longer-term survivors have been able to stop parenteral nutrition and resume normal diets.

Special tribute must be paid to the tremendous courage of the patients and their families who have participated in the clinical trials of small bowel transplantation. Each patient has enhanced our knowledge and helped to make this operation a worthwhile treatment. The potential of intestinal transplantation is most evident to those patients who have gained a healthy, normal lifestyle.

If the promising early results of FK 506 continue, transplantation of the small bowel will soon become the preferred treatment for chronic intestinal failure. At the present time the procedure is hampered by graft rejection, postoperative sepsis, lymphomas, and poor function. Further research is needed to develop protocols that will make small bowel transplantation safer and more reliable. Also, the cost effectiveness and quality of life provided by intestinal grafting will have to be closely monitored as the clinical indications expand.

DRG
RFMW

List of Contributors

Martin L Blakely MD, Division of Organ Transplantation, Harvard Medical School Department of Surgery, New England Deaconess Hospital, Boston, MA

R Randal Bollinger MD, PhD, Departments of Surgery and Immunology, Duke University Medical Center, Durham, NC

Nicole Brousse MD, Service de Pathologie, Hôpital Necker Enfants Malades, Paris

Bradley H Collins MD, Department of Surgery, Duke University Medical Center, Durham, NC

Olivier Goulet MD, PhD, Service de Gastroentérologie et Nutrition, Hôpital Necker Enfants Malades, Paris

Wuyi Xia MD, Department of Surgery, Brigham and Woman's Hospital, Harvard Medical School, Boston, MA

David R Grant MD, FRCSC, Multi-Organ Transplant Service, University Hospital, London, Ontario

Celia L Ingham Clark FRCS, Professorial Surgical Unit, St Bartholomew's Hospital, London

Kursheed N Jeejeebhoy MBBS, PhD, FRCP(C), University of Toronto Departments of Medicine and Nutrition, St Michael's Hospital, Toronto, Ontario

Barry D Kahan MD, PhD, Division of Immunology and Organ Transplantation, Department of Surgery, University of Texas Medical School, Houston, TX

Robert L Kirkman MD, Department of Surgery, Brigham and Woman's Hospital, Harvard Medical School, Boston, MA

Paul A Lear MS, FRCS, University of Bristol Department of Surgery, Southmead Hospital, Bristol

Vivian C McAlister FRCSC, FRCSI, Department of Surgery, Victoria General Hospital, Halifax, Nova Scotia, Canada

Anthony P Monaco MD, Division of Organ Transplantation, Harvard Medical School Department of Surgery, New England Deaconess Hospital, Boston, MA

Noriko Murase MD, Pittsburgh Transplant Institute and Department of Surgery, University of Pittsburgh Medical Center, Pittsburgh, PA

Yann Revillon MD, Service de Chirurgie Pediatrique, Hôpital Necker Enfants Malades, Paris

Claude Ricour MD, Service de Gastroentérologie et Nutrition, Hôpital Necker Enfants Malades, Paris

Wolfgang H Schraut MD, PhD, University of Pittsburgh, Pittsburgh, PA

Peter Schroeder Department of General Surgery, Gilead Hospital, Bielefeld, Germany

David Shaffer MD, Division of Organ Transplantation, Harvard Medical School Department of Surgery, New England Deaconess Hospital, Boston, MA

Thomas E Starzl MD, PhD, Pittsburgh Transplant Institute and Department of Surgery, University of Pittsburgh Medical Center, Pittsburgh, PA

Stanislaw M Stepkowski PhD, Division of Immunology and Organ Transplantation, Department of Surgery, University of Texas Medical School, Houston, TX

Satoru Todo MD, Pittsburgh Transplant Institute and Department of Surgery, University of Pittsburgh Medical Center, Pittsburgh, PA

Andreas Tzakis MD, Pittsburgh Transplant Institute and Department of Surgery, University of Pittsburgh Medical Center, Pittsburgh, PA

Richard F M Wood MD, FRCS, Professorial Surgical Unit, St Bartholomew's Hospital, London

1

Small bowel failure: causes and current treatment options

Kursheed N Jeejeebhoy

Management of intestinal failure

Definition of intestinal failure

Intestinal failure refers to the clinical effects of extensive small bowel injury. This injury results in inadequate absorption of solutes derived from the digested products of ingested food. Malabsorption of solute results in diarrhoea, fluid and electrolyte losses and malnutrition.

Physiological considerations

In order to understand the effects of intestinal resection it is important to review some essential aspects of gastrointestinal physiology.

Gastric emptying

The rate at which a meal enters the intestine is regulated by the rate of gastric emptying. Gastric emptying of liquids depends upon their osmolarity. For digestible solids the emptying is regulated by the particle size. However, of greater importance in relation to the short bowel syndrome is the fact that intestinal content entering the distal intestine inhibits gastric emptying.[1]

Small bowel

Small bowel motility is three times slower in the ileum than in the jejunum.[2] It is claimed that the ileocecal valve may slow transit although this is controversial.[3]

The small bowel receives about 5–6 litres of endogenous secretions and 2–3 litres of exogenous fluids per day. It reabsorbs most of this volume in the small bowel. The amount reabsorbed in the small intestine depends upon the nature of the meal.[4] With a meat and salad meal of low osmolality, most of the fluid is absorbed in the jejunum whereas with a milk and doughnut meal of high osmolality, less is absorbed proximally and more is absorbed distally. In addition, the absorptive processes are different in the jejunum as compared with the ileum. These differences depend partly on the nature of the electrolyte transport processes and partly on the permeability of the intercellular junctions. In general, water absorption is a passive process resulting from the active transport of nutrients and electrolytes. The transport of sodium creates an electrochemical gradient and also drives the uptake of sugars and amino acids across the intestinal mucosa. In addition, in the ileum there is neutral sodium chloride absorption. The net absorption depends not only upon these processes but upon the extent of back diffusion of the transported material into the intestinal lumen through 'leaky' intercellular junctions. In the jejunum these junctions are very leaky and jejunal contents are always isotonic. Fluid absorption in this region of the bowel is very inefficient when compared with the ileum. It has been estimated that the efficiency of water absorption is 44 per cent and 70 per cent of the ingested load in the jejunum and ileum respectively. For sodium the corresponding estimates are 13 per cent and 72 per cent.[5] Hence the ileum is important in the conservation of fluid and electrolytes.

Colon

The colon has the slowest transit varying between 24–150 hours. The intercellular junctions are tight in this part of the bowel and the efficiency of water and salt absorption in the colon exceeds 90 per cent.[5] In addition carbohydrate is fermented in the colon to short-chain fatty acids (SCFA) which in turn have two important actions. First, SCFA enhance salt and water absorption.[6] Second, the energy content of malabsorbed carbohydrates is salvaged by being absorbed as SCFA. Our recent data suggest that in short bowel patients this salvage may be greater than in normal bowel.[7] Thus the colon becomes an important organ for fluid and electrolyte conservation and for the salvage of malabsorbed energy substrates in patients with a short bowel.

Unique functions of the ileum

The ileum uniquely absorbs vitamin B_{12} and bile salts. Bile salts are essential for the efficient absorption of fats and fat soluble vitamins. Normally the demand for bile salts imposed by fat absorption cannot be met by synthesis alone. This full need is only met by ileal resorption of bile salts which are then recycled into the intestine. With ileal resection the loss of bile salts increases and is not met by an increase in synthesis. The bile salt pool is depleted and fat absorption is reduced. In addition loss of bile salts into the colon reduces the ability of the colon to reabsorb salt and water resulting in increased diarrhoea. In the colon bile salts are also dehydroxylated to deoxy bile salts which induce colonic water secretion.

Effects of intestinal resection

Motility

Gastric motility is enhanced by small bowel resection.[8] While proximal resection does not increase the rate of intestinal transit, ileal resection significantly accelerates intestinal transit[8,9]. In this condition the colon aids in slowing intestinal transit. In patients with a short bowel without a colon, an unabsorbable marker fed by mouth was completely excreted in a few hours.[10]

Absorption of fluid and electrolytes

The effect of intestinal resection on absorption depends upon the extent and site of resection. Proximal resection results in no bowel disturbance because the ileum and colon absorb the increased fluid and electrolyte load efficiently. The remaining ileum continues to absorb bile salts and thus there is little reaching the colon to impede salt and water resorption. In contrast when the ileum is resected, the colon receives a much larger load of fluid and electrolytes and also receives bile salts which reduce its ability to absorb salt and water, resulting in diarrhoea. In addition, if the colon is resected, the ability to maintain fluid and electrolyte homeostasis is severely impaired.[11]

Absorption of nutrients

Absorption of nutrients occurs throughout the small bowel and the removal of the jejunum alone results in the ileum taking over most of the lost function. In this situation there is no malabsorption.[12] In contrast even a loss of 100 cm of ileum causes steatorrhoea.[13] The degree of malabsorption increases with the length of resection and the variety of nutrients malabsorbed increases.[14,15] Balance studies of energy absorption showed that the absorption of fat and carbohydrate were equally reduced to between 50 and 75 per cent of intake.[16] However nitrogen absorption was reduced to a lesser extent namely to 81 per cent of intake. In the study of Ladefoged et al.,[15] the degree of calcium, magnesium, zinc, and phosphorus absorption was reduced but did not correlate with the remaining length of bowel and they recommended that in these patients parenteral nutrition was mandatory. Our studies showed a similar reduction in absorption but only half of the patients required parenteral replacement. The data taken as a whole suggest that it is easier to meet needs for energy and nitrogen by increasing oral intake than the needs for electrolytes and divalent ions. A review of the literature prior to the availability of parenteral nutrition shows that resections up to 33 per cent result in no malnutrition and those up to 50 per cent could be tolerated without special aids, but resections in excess of 75 per cent require nutritional support to avoid severe malnutrition.[17–27]

Complications of intestinal resection

Gastric hypersecretion and peptic ulceration

Gastric hypersecretion occurs immediately after intestinal resection and tends to be transient. However, in some patients peptic ulceration may occur. Treatment with H_2-blockers has been found to successfully heal the ulcer and reduce acid secretion.[28,29]

Cholelithiasis

After ileal resection there is interruption of the enterohepatic cycle of bile salts. In consequence bile salt loss occurs in excess of the ability of the liver to increase synthesis and the bile salt concentration in bile is reduced. The reduction of the concentration of chenodeoxycholate in the bile increases cholesterol secretion.[30] This combination makes the bile lithogenic. Clinically, in this situation an increased incidence of gallstones has been observed.[31] Recently a study in experimental animals has shown an increased incidence of pigment stones.[32]

Renal stones

Hyperoxaluria occurs in short bowel patients due to increased absorption of oxalate by the colon.[33] Bile salts in the colon increase oxalate absorption.[34] Hyperoxalauria is associated with renal stone formation and the propensity to form stones is reduced by reduced urinary citrate.[35] A low oxalate diet, cholestyramine to bind bile salts and an intake of citrate will prevent stone formation.

D-Lactic acidosis

In some patients with a short bowel a syndrome of slurred speech, ataxia, and altered affect may occur.[36] Superficially the patient appears 'drunk'. The cause of this syndrome is fermentation of malabsorbed carbohydrate in the colon to D-lactate and absorption of this metabolite.[37] The treatment of this condition involves the use of a low carbohydrate diet.[38]

Nutritional treatment

Based on the considerations discussed above, the approach to a patient with intestinal failure depends upon the extent of the intestinal loss or injury, the presence of continuing intestinal disease that reduces the functional length of the intestine and the site of resected bowel.

General therapeutic approaches

Initially an assessment should be made to determine whether the patient has had a resection which is unlikely to cause serious malabsorption, such as a jejunal resection leaving an intact ileum and colon. Such patients need observation and are likely to recover full bowel function without the need for nutritional or other therapeutic support. Others who have had a resection of less than 100 cm of terminal ileum will only require the use of a bile salt binder, cholestyramine 4–12 g per day to control bile salt-induced diarrhoea. The remaining patients with a greater length of resection should be treated as follows.

Initial treatment after resection

Control of diarrhoea

Diarrhoea is due to a combination of increased secretions, increased motility, and osmotic stimulation of water secretion due to malabsorption of luminal contents. Soon after resection, diarrhoea is controlled by restricting oral intake to reduce any osmotic component. Gastric hypersecretion can be controlled by the continuous infusion of 1200 mg of cimetidine per day. In addition, loperamide can be used to slow gastric and intestinal transit. If loperamide does not work then codeine or phenoxylate may be tried. However, these agents do not influence the small intestine and act by slowing gastric and colonic motility.

Intravenous fluids

In the immediate postoperative period all patients will require intravenous fluid and electrolytes to replace losses. Sodium and potassium chloride as well as magnesium are the most important ions to be replaced and plasma levels of these ions should be monitored frequently. Fluid is infused according to measured losses to maintain a urine output of about 2 litres per day. The infusion is tapered as oral intake is increased.

Oral feeding

The next consideration is to determine the nature of oral feeds. In patients who have more than 60–80 cm of bowel left, refeeding should be progressive with a view ultimately to a normal oral diet. By contrast in patients who have little small bowel left, the initial target should be small volume isotonic feeds containing a glucose-electrolyte content similar to the oral rehydration solution. The composition of this solution should be glucose 3.4 per cent with sodium 85–90 mM/l, potassium 12 mM/l, bicarbonate 9 mM/l and chloride 80–90 mM/l. Such a solution avoids osmotic stimulation of secretion and yet stimulates the bowel to absorb, thus promoting adaptation. For those having intermediate lengths of bowel progressive feeding should be attempted with the following plan. The same carbohydrate-electrolyte feeds as above should be started. A mixture of a similar composition has been shown to be well absorbed by patients with massive resection who have previously been dependent on intravenous fluids.[39] The diet should be lactose-free since lactase levels in such patients are reduced.[40] Vitamin B_{12} absorption should be measured and if subnormal injections of 200 μg per month should be started.

While it is popular to try defined formula diets in these patients, studies by McIntyre et al.[41] have shown that they are not absorbed better than a solid diet.

Early observations had suggested that a low fat diet with medium-chain triglyceride (MCT) and a high carbohydrate content was better for patients with a short bowel.[42–4] The theory behind these suggestions was the observation that malabsorbed long-chain triglyceride (LCT) can cause colonic water secretion resulting in higher faecal output with steatorrhoea, and consequently greater loss of divalent ions. However, such studies were not controlled and MCT can also cause osmotic diarrhoea. Using a controlled cross-over design in two studies[10,16] we have shown that a high fat diet was comparable to a high carbohydrate diet in regard to total fluid, energy, nitrogen, sodium, potassium and divalent ion absorption. We therefore recommend a low lactose diet containing high calories from both fat and carbohydrate and a high nitrogen intake. We aim to increase intake gradually to about 60 kcals/kg body weight to provide sufficient absorbed calories despite malabsorption. The rationale for this approach is discussed by Woolf et al.[16] In essence these patients malabsorb 50 per cent of their intake and by doubling the intake they absorbed sufficient calories for their daily needs. Supplements of potassium, magnesium, and zinc are given while monitoring serum levels. We recommend the gluconate and pyroglutamate form of zinc and magnesium because the sulphate form results in the ingestion an unabsorbable anion (sulphate) which will increase diarrhoea.

Parenteral nutrition

In patients with less than 60 cm of remaining small bowel and in those with a combined small bowel and colon resection parenteral nutrition is life-saving. It is started in such patients within a few days of the resection and initially 32 kcals/kg of a mixed energy substrate and 1 g/kg amino acids is infused with sodium 150–200 mM, potassium 60–100 mM, calcium 9–11 mM, magnesium 7–15 mM, and zinc 70–100 micromoles per day. Among trace elements, zinc is the most important as we have found large losses in patients with a high endogenous output of intestinal fluids. We recommend adding a basal amount of 5 mg/day to which is added 12 mg/L of diarrhoea + fistula + stomal losses. Oral feeds are simultaneously started and attempts are made to reduce parenteral feeding as oral feeds are increased. It will become apparent whether the patient needs parenteral feeding on a long-term basis. If that is the case then the patient should be started on a programme of home parenteral nutrition (HPN). We have found that as the bowel adapts over months and even years the patient requires less parenteral feeding. Ultimately in about 30 per cent of our patients HPN can be replaced by 2 litres of oral rehydration solution, high calorie diet and supplements of potassium, magnesium, calcium, fat soluble vitamins and zinc. They are monitored regularly until the weight is stable and they are in electrolyte balance. Hypomagnesemia is a particularly serious problem in these patients. Ingestion of magnesium salts orally enhances diarrhoea and therefore it often becomes difficult to use magnesium supplements orally. The author has successfully used Magnesium pyroglutamate for this purpose. This preparation is available as a palatable powder which is added to the gastrolyte supplement in quantities of 30 mM/d. If this approach is not successful then magnesium sulphate is injected intramuscularly in doses of 12 mM 1–3 times a week to supplement the oral intake.

Patients with even small amounts of residual bowel can absorb water soluble vitamins but have difficulty absorbing fat soluble vitamins. They require large doses of vitamin A, D and E to maintain normal levels. Pills often pass out whole in these patients, hence liquid preparations have to be used. The author recommends the measurement of vitamin levels and supplementation with aqueous preparations of vitamin A and E (Aqasol A and E) and 1,25 dihydroxy-vitamin D in doses which normalize the plasma levels. Normalization may not be possible with oral vitamins in some individuals especially vitamin E levels.

In others, an oral diet with intravenous fluid and electrolytes becomes necessary and in the remainder full parenteral nutrition is given.

Special considerations

Somatostatin analogue

Long-acting somatostatin analogue has become available and can be given subcutaneously in doses of 100 mg 3 times a day. All studies have shown a reduction in the volume of output and an increase in sodium or chloride absorption.[45–7] However, the reduction did not seem to be sufficient to avoid parenteral nutrition in patients who required it.[46]

Jejunal resection with intact ileum and colon

Patients in this category can be fed orally immediately and rarely have any problems.

Ileal resection of less than 100 cm with colon largely intact

Patients in this category have so-called choleraic diarrhoea, and are best helped by the administration of 4 g of cholestyramine three times a day to bind bile salts left unabsorbed by the resected ileum. Vitamin B_{12} absorption should be measured and if low should be injected intramuscularly in doses of 100 to 200 μg per month.

Ileal resection of more than 100 to 200 cm with colon largely intact

These patients have little difficulty in maintaining nutrition with an oral diet, but may have fatty acid diarrhoea. For such a patient fat restriction is mandatory. With the larger resection the bile salt pool is depleted and cholestyramine is no longer beneficial. Parenteral vitamin B_2 replacement is required.

Resection in excess of 200 cm of small bowel and lesser resection with associated colectomy

Patients of this class require the graduated adaptation programme indicated previously under general considerations.

Resection leaving less than 60 cm small bowel or only duodenum: massive bowel resection

Patients in this category need home parenteral nutrition indefinitely. However, many patients even in this category may show a surprising degree of adaptation and require less parenteral nutrition and benefit from orally absorbed nutrients. The indication to reduce parenteral nutrition is weight gain beyond the desired limit and the fact that reduced infusion does not cause electrolyte imbalance and dehydration.

Home parenteral nutrition (HPN)

This is a technique for providing all necessary nutrients intravenously at home to ambulatory patients with intestinal failure.

The team approach

This modality of treatment requires the services of physicians, nurses, pharmacists, dietitians, and social workers. Hence it is necessary to develop a team of such individuals to care for patients on HPN.

Venous access and infusion system

The patient needs to have an implanted central venous catheter which can be used for long periods. These catheters are made of silicone rubber and the tip is placed just above the right atrium. Catheters implanted high in the superior vena cava are prone to cause caval thrombosis. The catheter exits via a subcutaneous tunnel. Alternatively the catheter can be connected to a

of molecular structure on bile acid-induced alterations in absorptive function, permeability, and morphology in the perfused rabbit colon. *J Lab Clin Med* 1979; **94,** 661–74.
35. Pak CYC, Peterson R, Sakhaee K, Fuller C, Preminger G, Reisch J. Correction of hypocitraturia and prevention of stone formation by combined thiazide and potassium citrate therapy in thiazide-unresponsive hypercalciuric nephrolithiasis. *Am J Med* 1985; **79,** 284–8.
36. Traube M, Bock JL, Boyer JL. D-Lactic acidosis after jejunoileal bypass: identification of organic anions by nuclear magnetic resonance spectroscopy. *Ann Intern Med* 1983; **98,** 171–3.
37. Satoh T, Narisawa K, Konno T, Katoh T, Fujiyama J, Tomoe A, Metoki K, Hayasaka K, Tada K, Ishibashi M, Yamane N, Mitsuoka T, Benno Y. D-lactic acidosis in two patients with short bowel syndrome: bacteriological analyses of the fecal flora. *Eur J Pediatr* 1982; **138,** 324–6.
38. Ramakrishnan T, Stokes P. Beneficial effects of fasting and low carbohydrate diet in D-lactic acidosis associated with short-bowel syndrome. *J Parenter Enteral Nutr* 1985; **9,** 361–3.
39. Griffin GE, Fagan EF, Hodgson AJ, Chadwick VS. Enteral therapy in the management of massive gut resection complicated by chronic fluid and electrolyte depletion. *Dig Dis Sci* 1982; **27,** 902–8.
40. Richards AJ, Condon JR, Mallinson CN. Lactose intolerance following extensive small intestinal resection. *Br J Surg* 1971; **58,** 493–4.
41. McIntyre PB, Fitchew M, Lennard-Jones JE. Patients with a high jejunostomy do not need a special diet. *Gastroenterology* 1986; **91,** 25–33.
42. Andersson H, Isaksson B, Sjogren B. *Gut* 1974; **15,** 351–9.
43. Weser E. The management of patients after small bowel resection. *Gastroenterology* 1976; **71,** 146–50.
44. Zurier RB, Campbell RG, Hashim SA, Van Itallie TB. Use of medium-chain triglyceride in management of patients with massive resection of the small intestine. *N Engl J Med* 1966; **274,** 490–3.
45. Rodrigues CA, Lennard-Jones JE, Thompson DG, Farthing MJ. The effects of octreotide, soy polysaccharide, codeine and loperamide on nutrient, fluid and electrolyte absorption in the short-bowel syndrome. *Aliment Pharmacol Ther* 1989; **3,** 159–69.
46. Ladefoged K, Christensen KC, Hegnhoj J. *Gut* 1989; **30,** 943–9.
47. Dharmsathaphorn K, Gorelick FS, Sherwin RS, Cataland S, Dobbins JW, Somatostatin decreases diarrhea in patients with the short-bowel syndrome. *J Clin Gastroenterol* 1982; **4,** 521–4.
48. Jeejeebhoy KN. Enteral and parenteral nutrition. Civetta JM, Taylor RW, Kirby RR (eds) *Critical Care*. Philadelphia, PA, J.B. Lippincott, 1988, pp 513–34.
49. Shike M, Sturtridge WC, Tam CS, Harrison JE, Jones G, Murray TM, Husdan H, Whitwell J, Wilson DR, Jeejeebhoy KN. A possible role of vitamin D in the genesis of parenteral-nutrition-induced metabolic bone disease. *Ann Int Med* 1981; **95**(5), 560–8.
50. Langer B, McHattie JD, Zohrab WJ, Jeejeebhoy KN. Prolonged survival after complete small bowel resection using intravenous alimentation at home. *J Surg Res* 1973; **15**(3), 226–33.
51. Jeejeebhoy KN, Zohrab WJ, Langer B, Phillips MJ, Kuksis A, Anderson GH. Total parenteral nutrition at home for 23 months without complication and with good rehabilitation. A study of technical and metabolic features. *Gastroenterology* 1973; **65**(5), 811–20.
52. Detsky AS, McLaughlin JR, Abrams HB, L'Abbe KA, Whitwell J, Bombardier C, Jeejeebhoy KN. Quality of life of patients on long-term total parenteral nutrition at home. *J Gen Int Med* 1986; **1,** 26–33.

2

Experimental models of small bowel transplantation

Wolfgang H Schraut and Kenneth K W Lee

In the past two years small bowel transplantation has become a clinical reality in the form of protocolled trials. With any new form of medical/surgical therapy, early clinical experience is associated with new questions which need to find their answer in the experimental laboratory. Without doubt, the same holds true for small bowel transplantation. Against this background animal models of small bowel transplantation retain their significance as the main avenues to provide new information.

The experimental animal models come as large-animal (dog, pig, baboon) and small-animal (rat, mouse) models. At present, *ex vivo* culturing techniques using mucosal biopsies or enterocyte preparations are adjuncts to animal experimentation, but have not been utilized in lieu of whole organ transplantation *in vivo*.

Studies using large animals which, by mere size, seemingly simulate clinical practice more closely than rodents, are costly in terms of personnel, are very time consuming, require the utmost in supplies, demand specific experience and expertise in animal handling and, most of all, are conducted under the scrutiny and threatening/discouraging posture of animal rights activists and stringent regulations. One would expect that only large, well-staffed and well-funded research teams with lots of time would embark on large-animal studies in small bowel transplantation.

In the outset, studies using large animals, especially the dog, have provided the basic knowledge upon which all subsequent studies on small bowel transplantation expanded. Attempts at experimental small bowel transplantation date back to the beginning of the century. In 1901, E Ullmann reported to the Viennese Medical Society on his experiments with transplantation of intestinal segments, and in 1902, Alexis Carrel, who later received the Nobel Prize for medicine, published his studies in dogs. Major advances in small bowel transplantation were achieved in the early 1960s when numerous investigators, foremost among them Lillehei, documented the technical feasibility of small bowel transplantation in several animal models. Lillehei and his colleagues were the first to describe a technique for functional bowel transplantation in the dog.[1,2] These investigators replaced the entire small intestine of the recipient with a pedicle intestinal graft that required vascular anastomoses between the superior mesenteric artery and vein of the graft and the mesenteric vessels or, alternatively, the aorta and inferior vena cava of the recipient. The recipients of the orthotopic autografts survived indefinitely, whereas allografts were rejected within several days. Early studies performed with this model provided the experimental basis for the first 8 human small bowel transplants performed prior to the discovery of cyclosporin A, (CsA).

The effectiveness of various immunosuppressive regimens was evaluated in dog models involving transplantation of a small intestinal segment as a Thiry–Vella loop in the neck or abdomen, with anastomosis of the intestinal vessels either to the carotid artery and jugular vein or to the external iliac vessels, depending on the site of placement.[3–5] Similar studies were undertaken on pigs.[6,7] Orthotopic (graft in gastrointestinal continuity) and heterotopic transplantation models in dogs and pigs were also employed to develop methods of small bowel preservation,[8,9] and to establish methods for the monitoring of intestinal grafts subject to rejection (histomorphologic evaluation of graft biopsies,[10–12]) and to test the efficacy of CsA.[13–16] Many laboratories used large animals to train their team members in the technical aspects of transplantation preparing for human small bowel transplantation. Despite these unquestionably important advances achieved by experimentation on dogs and pigs, the large animal models are expected to be replaced by models using immunologically-defined inbred rodent species in the forseeable future.

In 1971, Monchik and Russell described the first rat model of small bowel transplantation.[17] In this model, microsurgical techniques are used to isolate and remove the donor small bowel based on a vascular pedicle consisting of the superior mesenteric artery with an attached aortic cuff in the fashion of Carrel, and the portal vein transected near its bifurcation. The graft is then revascularized by end-to-side anastomosis of the aortic cuff to the recipient's infrarenal aorta, and of the portal vein to the recipient's inferior vena cava, thereby establishing systemic venous outflow of the transplanted bowel. The ends of the transplanted bowel are exteriorized as abdominal wall stomas, creating a non-functional out-of-continuity Thiry–Vella loop. This model was used extensively to delineate the histopathologic course of rejection,[18,19] the clinical alterations and intestinal functional impairment associated with rejection,[20] and the course and alterations seen with graft-versus-host (GVH) disease induced by small bowel transplants.[21] Subsequently as orthotopic rat models with either porto-portal or portocaval venous anastomosis were described,[22,23] many studies previously done with heterotopic intestinal grafts were then repeated in the orthotopic model coming, in general, to the same results and conclusions. One of the disadvantages of the heterotopic model lies in the fact that during the early postoperative period and during rejection the bowel lumen becomes filled with mucous secretions which need to be irrigated out in order to prevent excessive dilatation.[24] Most likely, this occurs on account of disturbed motility coupled with the lack of chyme flow (bile, pancreatic secretions). Orthotopically placed grafts do not develop this complication by our experience. Furthermore, rejection of an orthotopically placed graft (whether by necrosis and/or fibrosis) invariably leads to the death of the recipient, a clear endpoint if one uses graft survival as a study parameter. In contrast, heterotopic intestinal grafts, especially segmental grafts, often become encapsulated and do not impair recipient survival; graft rejection under this circumstance is determined by the development of a palpable abdominal mass, a highly subjective approach.[25,26]

In our laboratory, we employ 4 separate models of small bowel transplantation in the rat which vary according to the route of venous outflow and placement of the graft with respect to the recipient's own small bowel. In addition to the model described by Monchik and Russell, which by convention is designated as systemic or caval venous outflow with heterotopic graft position, we have performed small bowel transplantation whereby the donor portal vein is anastomosed in end-to-side fashion to the recipient's portal vein, which directs venous outflow along its physiologic route. With either portal or systemic venous outflow, the graft may be positioned out of intestinal continuity, or heterotopically, or in intestinal continuity, or orthotopically, after resection of varying lengths of the recipient's own small intestine and completion of proximal and distal intestinal anastomoses. With orthotopic positioning and total or near total resection of the native small intestine, the recipient becomes nutritionally dependent upon the transplanted intestine. Orthotopic graft placement may be performed either at the time of graft revascularization or as a delayed second procedure. We favour orthotopic placement at the time of revascularization as little time is added to the surgical procedure and the added complication rate attributable to placement of the graft into intestinal continuity is small (5–10 per cent). This approach permits early study of graft function and avoids the need for a second major operative procedure with its potentially adverse impact on the rat. Institutional and external regulatory agency guidelines also increasingly restrict performance of multiple surgical procedures on the same experimental animal.

Other investigators have reported further modifications of the rat model of small bowel transplantation. Sonnino and Harmel[27] have described a model in which the superior mesenteric artery and vein are isolated within the small bowel mesentery. While this technique may more closely approximate the surgical approach for clinical small bowel transplantation, and although excellent results are reported using this technique, its advantages as an experimental model are unclear. Deltz and co-workers[28] have described a modified staged orthotopic procedure in which at the initial operation the distal end of the revascularized bowel is anastomosed in end-to-side fashion to the recipient's distal ileum and the proximal end is ligated. Resection of the recipient's own small bowel and proximal intestinal anastomosis are then performed 3 weeks later. Although excellent experimental results have also been reported using this model, its advantages over one-stage orthotopic intestinal transplantation are unclear. We use the Deltz model (first stage) presently to study various aspects of small bowel preservation. The main advantage over other heterotopic models lies in the fact that enterostomies are avoided. This, in turn, avoids the need to house rats individually so as to prevent stomal cannibalism. Furthermore, secretions from the transplant drain into the gastrointestinal tract and thus are not lost to the recipient. On the other hand of course, there is no direct access to the graft or direct visualization by the enterostoma.

For various genuine and perceived reasons, the results of large animal studies may be more directly applicable to human small bowel transplantation. To date, however, this remains more a theoretical than real advantage of these models. In contrast, the rat model of small bowel transplantation has provided several real advantages. Most important among these has been the ability to perform detailed immunologic studies. Using appropriately selected, well-defined, inbred strains of rats, immunologic responses following small bowel transplantation and the effectiveness of various immunosuppressive regimens for their control have been studied in the context of isolated rejection (F_1 hybrid to parental strain), isolated graft-versus-host disease (parental strain to F_1 hybrid; GVHD), and concurrent rejection and graft-versus-host disease (parental strain to fully allogeneic parental strain) with either graft rejection as the predominant event[29] or, when donor and/or host are pretreated, GVH-disease as the prominent development.[30] The availability of strain-specific monoclonal antibodies also permits investigations such as the repopulation of graft lymphoid tissues by recipient cells, and conversely, the trafficking of graft lymphoid tissue through the recipient.[31,32,33] These phenomena may have significant bearing on the preservation of the mucosal barrier function of the transplanted small intestine, as well as the development of GVHD following small bowel transplantation.

Because of size considerations, physiologic studies pertaining to small bowel transplantation have frequently been performed in large animal models. Advances in technology and methodology, however, increasingly allow these studies to be performed in the rat. Standard hematologic and serum chemistry measurements are easily obtained in the rat. The small samples obtainable from a rat are rarely limiting due to the great sensitivity of radioimmunoassay techniques. Absorption and ion flux studies using Ussing chambers,[34] and motility studies using miniaturized electrodes, can be performed in the rat following small bowel transplantation. With metabolic cages the intake of food and water can be accurately monitored, and metabolic studies such as nitrogen balance and faecal fat excretion can be easily completed.[35] With newer instrumentation, endoscopic examination of transplanted rat small intestine is now possible. These and other advances continue to diminish the technical advantages of large animal models over the rat model for physiologic studies.

The rat models of small bowel transplantation offer several practical advantages over either the dog or pig models. The operative procedure can be easily mastered by individuals having no prior surgical experience within a short time and, in contrast to the large animal, procedures can be performed by a single individual with no assistants. Once mastered, the procedure can be performed quickly with a high technical success rate. One-stage orthotopic small bowel transplantation requires 1¾ to 2½ hours from the start of the donor procedure to the completion of the implantation procedure, and an overall technical success rate of 80 to 90 per cent has been reported. The postoperative care of rats undergoing small bowel transplantation is also simple in comparison to dogs or pigs. Perioperative intravenous fluid administration is not necessary in the rat. Immediately following transplantation, water can be given orally and after two days a regular diet of laboratory chow can be resumed even in rats undergoing orthotopic transplantation. The incidence of intra-abdominal or incisional infection is extremely low, avoiding the need for perioperative antibiotic therapy. Immunosuppressive medications or other drugs can be conveniently administered by subcutaneous or intramuscular injection or by gavage.

From a cost perspective, the rat model offers additional advantages over the dog and pig models. The complete instrumentation necessary to perform small bowel transplantation in the rat costs less than $US600. An operating microscope adds substantially to this cost but is unnecessary; we have found that optical visors costing less than $US40 each provide adequate magnification for the microsurgical procedures. Operating loupes are another less expensive alternative to an operating microscope.

The purchase and housing of animals contribute enormously to the overall cost of small bowel transplantation research and further favour use of the rat model. In our institution, a donor-recipient pair of inbred rats costs about $US30, and other necessary materials such as suture cost less than $US20. In contrast, a donor-recipient pair of dogs costs about $US600. Use of the experimental surgery suite as required for large animal experiments, but not rat experiments adds about $US200 per experiment. The daily charge for animal care is less that $US0.50 for rats, and more than $US7.50 for dogs. The cost of an experimental group of 6 transplanted dogs followed for 6 months may thus approach $US13,000, in comparison to $US600 for a group of 6 rats.

Finally, societal concerns and pressures are leading to increasing restrictions upon the use of animals in research. While societal pressures and institutional regulations will undoubtedly evolve, at present fewer restrictions apply to the use of rats in research. Because of these considerations, rat models of small bowel transplantation have been adopted by most laboratories engaged in small bowel transplantation research.

Rats are particularly suited for this purpose because much of our knowledge on gastrointestinal physiology metabolism, immunology, and anatomy has been developed through experimentation on rodents. Our laboratory has used the rat model for the past 10 years, accumulating long and large experiences with this model (Table 2.1).

We have studied the function of small bowel transplants when the absence of graft rejection and GVHD is ensured by use of highly inbred syngeneic donor-recipient strain combinations. Following one-stage orthotopic small bowel transplantation with physiologic portal venous outflow in the syngeneic Lewis (LEW) to LEW rat strain combination, no differences between transplant recipients and normal controls with respect to survival, weight gain, serum protein, albumin, cholesterol, or triglyceride levels, or uptake of intraluminal glucose or maltose can be detected.[36] The LEW to LEW strain combination has also been useful for determination of the nutritional and metabolic consequences of directing venous outflow of the graft into the systemic rather than portal circulation. Following orthotopic transplantation with venous outflow into the inferior vena cava, none of the above parameters differ significantly from normal controls or transplant recipients with portal venous outflow. Despite the partial mesocaval shunt which results from systemic venous outflow of the transplanted small bowel, the serum ammonia levels of fasted transplant recipients do not differ significantly from controls. Fed transplant recipients with systemic venous outflow, however, do have alterations in levels of selected amino acids and significantly elevated serum ammonia levels, although these levels are markedly less than those observed after total portocaval shunting and are not associated with any gross behavioural abnormalities in the rats.[23,36,37]

Using the rat model we have also studied the influence of venous drainage on allograft rejection.[29] Heterotopic transplantation in the Lewis × Brown Norway (BN) F_1 (LBN F_1) to LEW unidirectional rejection strain combination results in two distinct patterns of graft rejection which are dependent upon the route of venous outflow. Systemic venous outflow results in acute rejection leading to graft destruction and recipient death after a mean survival of 11.8 ± 0.45 days. Portal venous outflow results in less fulminant rejection that follows a more prolonged course. Graft destruction eventually ensues but is often associated with graft encapsulation and recipient survival. These findings suggest that portal venous outflow of transplanted small bowel is not only more physiologic, but also confers immunologic advantages. Studies with other vascularized organ allografts have demonstrated a similar benefit of portal venous outflow. This effect appears minor, however, and is not seen when orthotopic small bowel transplantation is performed: acute rejection with no differences in recipient survival ensues irrespective of the type of venous drainage.[25] Shaffer et al. have also failed to observe any survival benefit when orthotopic transplantation is performed with portal venous outflow.[36]

The study of immunologic reactions which develop following small bowel transplantation is possible with the availability of highly inbred rat strains. In addition to eliciting a typical host

Table 2.1 Summary of selected experimental studies

Donor	Recipient	Treatment/model	Observation
LEW	LEW	Portal outflow	Physiologically equivalent to normal rat
		Systemic outflow	Partial mesocaval shunt results in elevated ammonia level in fed rats but otherwise produces few physiologic abnormalities
LBN F_1	LEW	Heterotopic with systemic outflow	Acute rejection leading to recipient death
		Heterotopic with portal outflow	Delayed course of acute rejection often allowing recipient survival despite graft loss
LEW	LBN F_1	—	Fatal GVHD
		1000 rad *in vitro* irradiation of graft	No GVHD, long-term recipient survival, normal graft function
BN	LEW	Orthotopic with no immunosuppression	Acute rejection leading to recipient death
		CsA 15 mg/kg IM d. 0–4	Delayed course of acute rejection leading to recipient death. Survival prolonged (MST = 24.3 ± 3.9 d.)
		CsA 15 mg/kg IM d. 0–6	Subacute/chronic rejection with occasional long-term survival
		CsA 15 mg/kg IM d. 0–6 then QOD to d. 28	Long-term survival of all graft recipients
		FK 506 2 mg/kg IM d. 0–4	Long-term survival of all graft recipients
BN	LEW	CsA 10 mg/kg IM d. 0–4	Acute rejection leading to recipient death. Slight prolongation of survival (MST = 16.5 ± 2.3 d.)
		CsA 10 mg/kg IM 0–4 plus FK 506 2 mg/kg d. 14,16,18	Graft 'rescue' with long-term survival, restoration of graft histology, and recovery of graft function
ACI	LEW	—	Acute rejection (MST = 7.2 ± 0.7 d.)
ACI	LEW	CsA 15 mg/kg IM d. 0–6 then QOD to d. 28	Macroscopic and microscopic signs of chronic rejection (MST = 130.3 ± 66.1 d.)
		CsA 15 mg/kg IM d. 0–6 then QOD to d. 28 plus FK 506 2 mg/kg day for 5 d. or CsA 15 mg/kg/d QOD for 28 days	Rescue treatment started with clinical signs of chronic rejection (day 60–90). Progression of chronic rejection temporarily halted

response (host versus graft = rejection), the small bowel graft, by virtue of its large content of immunologically competent lymphoid cells present in the mesenteric lymph nodes, Peyer's patches, and bowel wall, can mediate a graft-versus-host response or even lethal GVHD. The significance of GVHD following clinical small bowel transplantation is still uncertain, possibly even of no concern. Nevertheless, unidirectional GVHD following experimental small bowel transplantation can be studied using the LEW to LBN F_1 strain combination.[21] In this model, GVHD leads to recipient death after a mean survival of 14.0 ± 0.7 days (orthotopic position). The clinical findings typical of GVHD arising from other causes are present: progressive weight loss, diarrhoea, alopecia, and dermatitis. Pathologic findings are also typical of GVHD: severe enteritis affecting the recipient's native small bowel but sparing the transplanted bowel develops; recipient lymph nodes and spleen exhibit marked decreases in cellularity, particularly in the germinal follicles and white pulp areas, and loss of normal histologic architecture; prominent splenomegaly with a significantly increased spleen:body weight ratio evolves; epidermal hyperkeratosis and cutaneous infiltration by mononuclear and polymorphonuclear cells occurs.

This and other parent to F_1 hybrid rat strain combinations have been used not only to characterize GVHD, but also to design methods to prevent its development. These have included methods which reduce the mass of lymphoid tissue transferred, such as surgical excision of the graft mesenteric lymph nodes,[38,39] shortening of graft length,[38] and donor pretreatment with anti-

A, Jehannin B, Ghnassia D, Duval C, Ghnassia J-c, Jos J, Fontaine J-L, Navarro J, Schmitz J, Gallix P. Conversation hypothermique et autotransplantation du l'intestin grêle chez le porchelet. *Gastroenterol Clin Bio* 1981; **5,** 977–86.

9. Raju S, Fujiwara H, Lewin JR, Grogan JB. Twelve-hour and twenty four-hour preservation of small bowel allografts by simple hypothermia. *Transplantation* 1988; **45,** 290–3.
10. Stauffer UG, Mona D, Schmerline DH. Monitoring of small bowel transplants by sequential mucosal suction biopsies. *Z Kinderchir Grenzeb* 1975; **16,** 32–7.
11. Cohen Z, Nordgren S. Lossing A et al. Morphological studies of intestinal allograft rejection. Immunosuppression with cyclosporine. *Dis Colon Rectum* 1984; **27,** 228–34.
12. Millard PR, Dennison A, Hughes DA et al. Morphology of intestinal allograft rejection and the inadequacy of mucosal biopsy in its recognition. *Br J Exp Pathol* 1986; **67** 1, 687–98.
13. Ricour C, Revillon Y, Arnaud-Battandier F, Ghnassia D, Weyne P, Lauffenburger A, Jos J, Fontaine JL, Gallix P, Vaiman M. Successful small bowel allografts in piglets using cyclosporine. *Transplant Proc* 1983; **XV,** 4, Supp 1.
14. Diliz-Perez HS, McClure, J, Bedetti C, Hong HQ, Santibanes ED, Shaw BW, Van Thiel D, Iwatsuki S, Starzl TE. Successful small bowel allotransplantation in dogs with cyclosporine and prednisone. *Transplantation* 1984; **37,** 126–9.
15. Fujiwara H, Raju S, Grogan JB et al. Total orthotopic small bowel allotransplantation in the dog. *Transplantation* 1987; **44,** 747–53.
16. Grant D, Duff J, Zhong R et al. Successful intestinal transplantation in pigs treated with cyclosporine. *Transplantation* 1988; **45,** 279.
17. Monchik GJ, Russell PS. Transplantation of small bowel in the rat: technical and immunological considerations. *Surgery* 1971; **70,** 693–702.
18. Madara JL, Kirkman RL. Structural and functional evolution of jejunal allograft rejection in rats and the ameliorating effects of cyclosporine therapy. *J Clin Invest* 1985; **75,** 502–12.
19. Rosemurgy AS, Schraut WH. Small-bowel allografts: Sequence of histologic changes in acute and chronic rejection. *Am J Surg* 1986; **151,** 470–5.
20. Billiar T, Garberoglio C, Schraut WH. Maltose absorption as an indicator of small intestinal allograft rejection. *J Surg Res* 1984; **37,** 75.
21. Schraut WH, Lee KKW, Dawson PJ, Hurst RD. Graft-versus-host disease induced by small bowel allografts. *Transplantation* 1986; **41,** 286–90.
22. Kort WJ, Westkroeck DL, MacDicken I et al. Orthotopic total small-bowel transplantation in the rat. *Eur Surg Res* 1973; **5,** 81–9.
23. Schraut WH, Abraham VS, Lee KKW. Portal versus caval venous drainage of small bowel allografts: technical and metabolic consequences. *Surgery* 1986; **99,** 193–8.
24. Schraut WH, Rosemurgy AS, Riddel RM. Prolongation of intestinal allograft survival without immunosuppressive drug therapy. *J Surg Res* 1983; **34,** 597–60.
25. Lee KKW, Schraut WH. Small-bowel transplantation in the rat. Graft survival with heterotopic vs. orthotopic position. In Deltz E, Thiede A, Hamelmann H (eds) *Small-bowel transplantation. Experimental and clinical fundamentals*. Heidelberg, Springer-Verlag, pp. 7–13, 1986.
26. Grant D, Zhong R, Hurlbut D, Garcia B, Chen H, Lamont D, Wang P, Stiller C, Duff J. A comparison of heterotopic and orthotopic intestinal transplantation in rats. *Transplantation* 1991; **51,** 948–54.
27. Sonnino RE, Harmel RP. Technical aspects of intestinal transplantation in the rat. *J Invest Surg* 1988; **1,** 55–64.
28. Deltz E, Thiede A. Experimental transplantation of small intestine. Microsurgical techniques and their applicability in research. In Olszewsky W (ed.) *Handbook of Microsurgery. 2*. Boca Raton, FL: CRC Press, pp. 419–29, 1984.
29. Schraut WH, Abraham VS, Lee KKW. Portal versus systemic venous drainage for small-bowel allografts. *Surgery* 1985; **98,** 579–85.
30. Langrehr JM, Hoffman RA, Banner B, Stangl MJ, Monyhan H, Lee KKW, Schraut WH. Induction of graft-*versus*-host disease and rejection by sensitized small bowel allografts. *Transplantation* 1991; **52,** 399–405.
31. Murase N, Demetris AJ, Matsuzaki T, Yagihasi A, Todo S, Fung J, Starzl TE. Long survival in rats after multivisceral versus isolated small bowel allotransplantation under FK 506. *Surgery* 1991; **110,** 87–98.
32. Langrehr JM, Hoffman RA, Demetris AJ, Lee KKW, Neuhaus P, Wren SM, Ildstad ST, Schraut WH. Evidence that indefinite survival of small bowel allografts achieved by a brief course of cyclosporine or FK 506 is not due to systemic hyporesponsiveness. *Transplantation* 1992; **54,** 505.
33. Langrehr JM, Demetris AJ, Banner B, Lee TK, Müller AR, Lee KKW, Schraut WH. Mucosal recipient-type mononuclear repopulation and low-grade chronic rejection occurs simultaneously in indefinitely surviving recipients of small bowel allografts. *Transplant International* (in press).
34. Lee TK, Cardona MA, Kurkchubasche AG, Smith SD, Müller AR, Lee KKW, Rowe MI, Schraut WH. Mucosal glutamine utilization after small-bowel transplantation: An electrophysiologic study. *J Surg Res* 1992; **52,** 605–14.
35. Langrehr JM, Reilly MJ, Banner B, Warty VS, Lee KKW, Schraut WH. Hepatic steatosis due to total parenteral nutrition: The influence of short-gut syn-

drome, refeeding and small bowel transplantation. *J Surg Res* 1991; **50,** 335–43.
36. Lee KKW, Schraut WH. Structure and function of orthotopic small-bowel allografts in rats treated with cyclosporine. *Am J Surg* 1986; **151,** 55–60.
37. Shaffer D, Diflo T, Love W, Clowes GHA, Maki T, Monaco AP. Immunologic and metabolic effects of caval versus portal venous drainage in small-bowel transplantation. *Surgery* 1988; **104,** 518–24.
38. Deltz E, Ulrich K, Schack T, Friedrichs B, Muller-Ruchholtz W, Muller-Hermelink HK, Thiede A. Graft-*versus*-host reaction in small bowel transplantation and possibilities for its circumvention. *Am J Surg* 1986; **151,** 379–86.
39. Luck R, Klempnauer J, Steiniger B. Abrogation of lethal graft-versus-host disease in MHC disparate small-bowel transplantation in the rat by mesenteric lymphadenectomy. *Transplant Proc* 1990; **22,** 2471.
40. Shaffer D, Maki T, DeMichele SJ, Karlstad MD, Bistrian BR, Balogh K, Monaco AP. Studies in small bowel transplantation. Prevention of graft-*versus*-host disease with preservation of allograft function by donor pretreatment with antilymphocyte serum. *Transplantation* 1988; **45,** 262–9.
41. Deaton DH, Barker CF, Naji A. Effect of selective depletion of donor $CD8^+$ lymphocytes on graft-*versus*-host disease in small-bowel transplantation. *Transplant Proc* 1990; **22,** 2467–8.
42. Deltz E, Ulrichs K, Engemann R, Schack T, Friedrichs B, Muller-Ruchholtz W, Muller-Hermelink HK, Thiede A. Prevention of graft-*versus*-host reaction following small bowel transplantation by temporary cyclosporine treatment. *Transplant Proc* 1983; **15,** 3027–31.
43. Hoffman AL, Makowka L, Banner B, Cai X, Cramer DV, Pascualone A, Todo S, Starzl TE. The use of FK 506 for small intestine allotransplantation. *Transplantation* 1990; **49,** 483–90.
44. Lee KKW, Schraut WH. In vitro allograft irradiation prevents graft versus host disease in small-bowel transplantation. *J Surg Res* 1985; **38,** 364–72.
45. Sigalet DL, Kneteman NM, Fedorak RN, Kizilisik AT, Thomson ABR. Intestinal function following allogeneic small intestinal transplantation in the rat. *Transplantation* 1992; **53,** 264.
46. Lee KKW, Langrehr JM, Stangl MJ, Wachs M, Schraut WH. Successful treatment of ongoing graft rejection permits recovery of graft structure and function. *Surgical Forum* 1990; **00,** 410–12.
47. Lee KKW, Stangl MJ, Todo S, Langrehr JM, Starzl TE, Schraut WH. Successful orthotopic small bowel transplantation with short term FK 506 immunosuppressive therapy. *Transplant Proc* 1990; **22**(Suppl. 1), 78–9.
48. Murase N, Demetris AJ, Kim DG, Todo S, Fung JJ, Starzl TE. Rejection of multivisceral allografts in rats: a sequential analysis with comparison to isolated orthotopic small bowel and liver grafts. *Surgery* 1990; **108,** 880–9.
49. Schraut WH, Lee KKW, Sitrin M. Recipient growth and nutritional status following transplantation of segmental small-bowel allografts. *J Surg Res* 1987; **43,** 1–9.
50. Sonnino RE, Teitelbaum DH, Dunaway DJ, Harmel RP. Small bowel transplantation permits survival in rats with lethal short-gut syndrome. *J Ped* 1989; **24,** 959.
51. Goulet O, Revillon Y, Jan D, Brousse N, De Potter S, Cerf-Bensussan N, Rambaud C, Buisson C, Pellerin D, Mougenot JF, Fischer A, Ricour C. Small-bowel transplantation in children. *Transplant Proc* 1990; **22,** 2499–500.
52. Todo S, Tzakis A, Abu-Elmagd K, Ryes J et al. Intestinal transplantation in composite visceral grafts or alone. *Ann Surg* 1992; **216,** 223.
53. Grant D, Wall W, Mimeault R, Zhong R, Ghent C, Garcia B, Stiller C, Duff J. Successful small-bowel/liver transplantation. *Lancet* 1990; **335,** 181.
54. Langrehr JM, Lee KKW, Wachs ME, Lee TK, Stangl MJ, Venkataramanan R, Kunz HW, Schraut WH. Comparison of the effectiveness of cyclosporine A in small-bowel transplantation using different rat strain combinations. *Transplant Proc* 1990; **22,** 2533–5.
55. Langrehr JM, Banner B, Lee KKW, Schraut WH. Clinical course, morphology and treatment of chronically rejecting small bowel allografts. *Transplantation* 1993; 55, 242–50.

3

The physiology of transplanted small intestine

Paul A Lear

Introduction

Physiological studies of transplanted small intestine have been severely hampered by the lack of a selective and potent immunosuppressant which could prevent rejection of the graft.[1,2] The introduction of the undecapeptide cyclosporin A has gone a long way in providing new information on function of allografted bowel, under conditions of immune quiescence. Prior to the introduction of cyclosporin there were only short-term physiological studies on allografts and the reproducible experimental data was largely based on autotransplants.[3,4] Allografts in recipients receiving conventional immunosuppression were inevitably undergoing a degree of rejection and physiological studies need to be interpreted in that light. Much of the information from autotransplantation is highly relevant, because under ideal immunological conditions allografts should behave as autografts. It is fortunate that using inbred rodent strains, isografts have been available for study under a variety of experimental circumstances. These include the full-length accessory heterotopic isograft which would otherwise be a serious missing link between allografts and autotransplants.

Many satisfactory immunosuppressive regimens using cyclosporin have been established in rodent small bowel transplant models enabling detailed and reproducible short-term and long-term studies on graft physiology.[5,6,7,8] The success in larger animal models has been more sporadic and chronic rejection has been a complicating feature. The data in dogs, pigs and primates therefore reflect broad concepts, and confirmation of the relevance of the results found in small animals, rather than providing precise detail.[9,10,11]

Transplantation

The process of transplantation disturbs intestinal physiology in a variety of ways. Anatomical changes include permanent disruption of the extrinsic autonomic nerve supply and temporary loss of formal lymphatic drainage. Ischaemic damage which causes mucosal dysfunction is variable and the recovery takes place between two and five days.[12,13] Severe mucosal damage results in loss of barrier function and the potential lethal complication of endotoxaemia.[14] Graft placement into an accessory heterotopic position results in the loss of luminal nutrition[15,16,17] and provides a haven for opportunist and potentially pathogenic bacteria.[18] The choice of venous drainage has implications for immunological responses and the partial porto-systemic shunting of absorbed nutrients.[19,20,21] Immunological rejection complicates all these issues and occurs at a time when the graft is recovering from surgery and adapting to new environmental demands.

A wide variety of immunological and anatomical models of intestinal transplantation has enabled investigators to define the different roles of these factors and their influence on graft function. This chapter reviews intestinal absorption and physiology and outlines the problems which have been encountered following small bowel transplantation. The ability of transplants to support growth and metabolism is discussed. Finally, the effects of transplantation on gut coordination and motility are considered.

Digestion and absorption – physiology in normal intestine

The macromolecular components of food are hydrolysed by digestive enzymes. This splitting process produces amino acids from proteins, monosaccharides from carbohydrates, and fatty acids and glycerine from fats. It is in this fashion that they are absorbed. The breakdown of proteins is particularly important to prevent direct absorption and immunological sensitization to foreign material.

Enzymes involved in the breakdown of oligosaccharides and oligopeptides are located on the surface of enterocytes. The luminal surface is composed of a brush-border of microvilli. The brush-border contains membrane-bound enzyme of both enterocyte and pancreatic origin. Putative active transport systems exist within the cell membrane, adjacent to the enzymes and are responsible for nutrient absorption. Enterocytes have a high turnover rate, originating within the crypts and migrating along the villus and finally being shed into the lumen within a few days. The shed enterocytes release membrane-bound enzymes and are themselves digested and, for the most part, reabsorbed.

The small intestine plays a prime role in the absorptive process. The surface area amounts to 200 m^2 in humans, and much of the surface amplification is due to the microvilli. Blood flow through the intestine varies with digestive phases. Considerable shunting occurs during the resting phase resulting in a lower mucosal blood flow when compared to active digestion.

Absorption is the net transport from the luminal to the serosal side of the enterocyte. The basic events include both passive (diffusion/osmosis) and active, energy-consuming transport mechanisms. Substances which move by diffusion and osmosis include water, chloride, and certain vitamins. The high lipid component of the cell membrane demands a degree of fat solubility for substances to diffuse. The protein and carbohydrate components of food are absorbed by active transport mechanisms.

Proteins and polypeptides are broken down by exo- and endopeptidases of mainly brush-border or pancreatic origin. Whole protein is only absorbed by neonates; thereafter amino acids and oligopeptides are taken up by stereo-specific (L amino acids are preferred), Na^+-dependent, active transport systems in the enterocyte membrane. There are four discrete systems for neutral amino acids, basic amino acids, immuno acids and glycine, and finally dicarbonic acids.

Carbohydrates comprise chiefly of glucose in the form of long chains with α 1,4 glycosidic bonds (amylose) and 1.6 linked branch chains (amylopectin). The former is broken down by saliva and pancreatic amylase. The amylopectin is split at the brush-border. Specific brush-border disaccharidases break down simple sugars to monosaccharides. Na^+-dependent carrier transport occurs for sugars such as galactose and glucose. Mannose and pentose diffuse across while fructose is absorbed by facilitated diffusion.

Fats are chiefly digested by a pancreatic lipase, phospholipase and cholesterol hydrolase. Brush-border lipase activity is unimportant. Short- and intermediate-chain fatty acids diffuse directly into the enterocytes. Long-chain fatty acids and cholesterol mix with bile salts to form micelles which enter the spaces between the microvilli and are transferred into the enterocyte membrane. Within the enterocyte the fat fragments are reassembled into triglycerides, cholesterol, and phospholipids and converted to lipoproteins, chylomicrons, and very low-density lipoprotein before being released into the lymphatics. The process is extremely efficient and in humans the daily excretion of fat is only 6 g, 3 g of which is accounted for by shed epithelial cells and bile.[22]

Water and electrolytes move in both directions within the small intestine and these shifts maintain isotonicity between luminal content and plasma. When osmotically active particles are absorbed during digestion, water follows along the osmotic gradient. The main site of water and salt absorption is the upper jejunum. There is a large capacity for the nervous system to influence ion and water transport. Not only do sensory receptors within the gut wall continually monitor the luminal activity and transmit the information to the integrated circuitry of the ganglia, but some sensory information is also processed within the central nervous system. Impulses for effector functions are relayed via the autonomic sympathetic and parasympathetic nerves.[23–26] Extra-

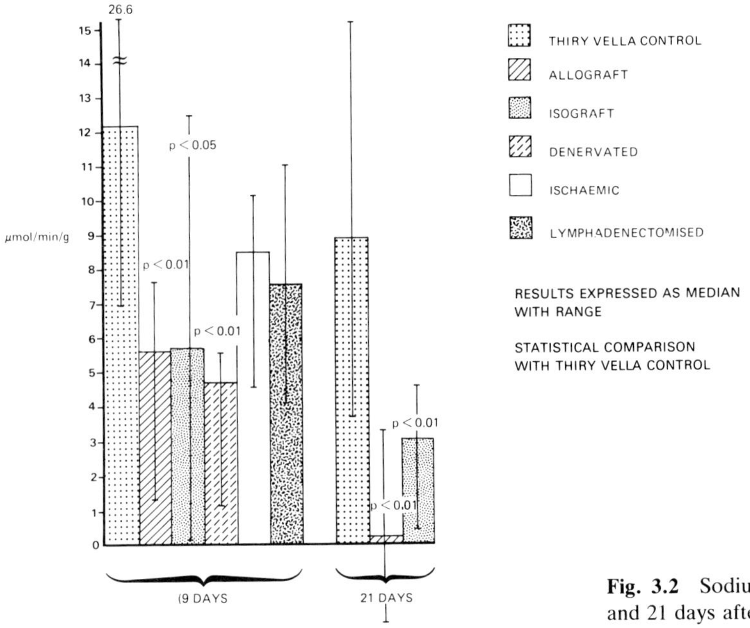

Fig. 3.2 Sodium absorption from glucose saline solution 9 and 21 days after transplantation.

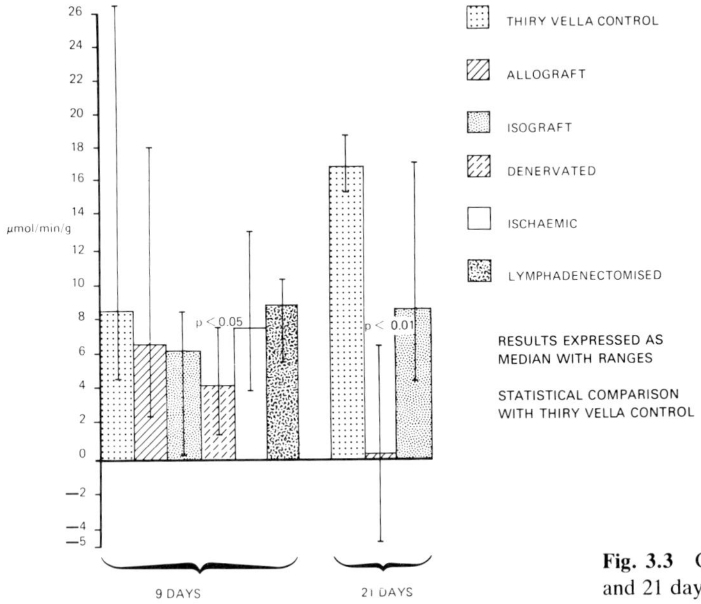

Fig. 3.3 Chloride absorption from glucose saline solution 9 and 21 days after transplantation.

the mucosa of grafts transplanted into a heterotopic position for 35 days.[50] This caused a significant diminution in the villous surface area. The *in vivo* absorption of water was reduced when correlated with graft length, but careful analysis showed that the absorption was increased when corrected for surface area. When heterotopic grafts were placed in orthotopic continuity in longer-term studies (56 days) a considerable degree of adaptation occurred particularly in ileal mucosa where the villi appear to hyperregenerate. Correspondingly, there is an increase in water absorption to supra-normal levels, and this related to graft length as well as surface area.

Carbohydrate absorption

Glucose and maltose absorption have been studied more extensively than any other nutrient and have been promoted as markers of immunological damage to the graft.[11,19,20,33,37,47,51,52] It is remarkable that there is uniform agreement that absorption of these simple sugars is very comparable to that of normal bowel in most experimental settings, including autotransplants and adequately immunosuppressed allografts, even when grafts are placed in a heterotopic position (Fig. 3.4). There is also conformity in the view that rejection is accompanied by an early deterioration in absorptive capacity, although studies carried out in animals using conventional immunosuppression with azathioprine and steroids were concerned with leakage of glucose across a 'semi-permeable' barrier caused by ongoing rejection.[53] Overall opinion would now suggest immunological damage would need to be very advanced for this to be tenable, and fluid loss from plasma into rejecting bowel would give rise to a moderate hyperglycaemia.

Studies of the rate of radiolabelled glucose absorption in heterotopic canine intestine show peaks of serum activity after 5 minutes in autotransplants compared with 10 minutes in nonrejecting allografts and 15 minutes in rejecting grafts. Peak activity was significantly reduced in the rejecting grafts compared to the other groups.[34]

There is a single study in primates which has taken a multifaceted approach to carbohydrate absorption.[11] Monosaccharides (dextrose and zylose), disaccharides (sucrose and maltose) and the polysaccharide Progestemil (containing corn syrup and tapioca starch) have individually been assessed for their absorptive capacity by heterotopic allografts between 12 and 70 days posttransplantation. All these carbohydrates appeared to be well absorbed.

Allied to carbohydrate absorption has been the immunohistochemical analysis of brush-border enzymes within the graft enterocytes.[54] The identification of early loss of intracytoplasmic maltase from these brush-border cells during rejection suggests that maltose absorption may be a better physiological marker to assess immunological damage than the use of xylose or glucose.[9,53]

Amino acids

From the introductory paragraphs, it is clear that the mechanisms of amino acid absorption are varied. Few studies have incorporated reports on absorption profiles[7,35] and these appear to reflect glucose uptake, which is compatible with the

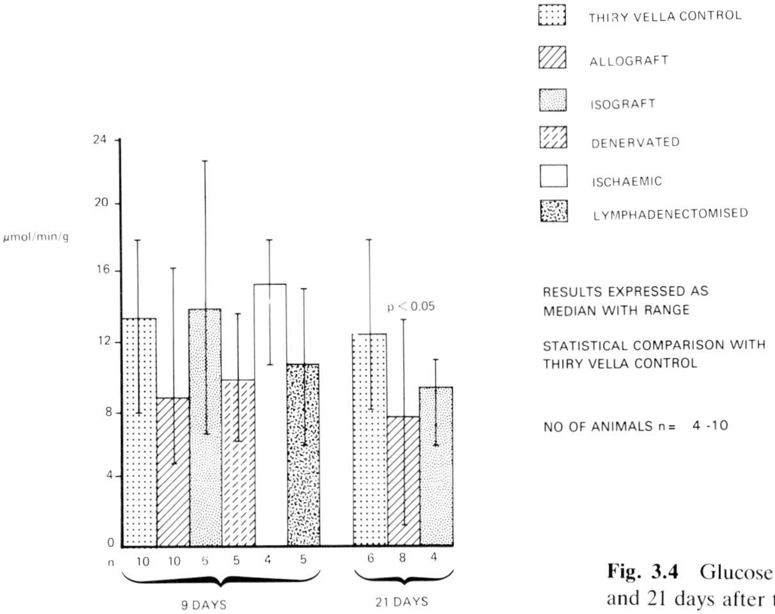

Fig. 3.4 Glucose absorption from glucose saline solution 9 and 21 days after transplantation.

common pathway of Na$^+$-dependent transport mechanisms. The importance of such amino acids as glutamine and alanine for local enterocyte nutrition cannot be over-emphasized and will putatively be incorporated into protocols involving heterotopic grafting.

Lymphatic regeneration and fat absorption

It is logical to couple the absorption of fat with the regeneration of formal lymphatic drainage of the grafted intestine. During the process of transplantation the lymphatics are disrupted. In the early postoperative phase any lymph drains freely into the peritoneal cavity and is gradually absorbed by that surface. Several groups have investigated regeneration of lymphatics after autotransplantation of the intestine by observing either dye directly crossing the mesenteric suture line, following its subserosal injection, or by the injection of X-ray opaque material into the mesenteric lymphoid tissue of the graft.[55] The first signs of true lymphatic regeneration occur at about two weeks after transplantation in the autotransplanted animals. In lymphangiography studies it would appear that significant channels to carry the contrast material are not present until about 3 to 4 weeks postoperatively.[56] In earlier studies using conventional immunosuppression it was not possible to achieve a sufficient length of allograft survival to demonstrate neolymphatic drainage.

A recent study between isografted Lewis rats has shown that there is a small degree of primitive lymphatic drainage as early as 3 days after grafting.[57] Clusters of chylomicrons and long-chain fatty acids could be seen within the retroperitoneum of the recipient. However, cyclosporin appeared to delay the regeneration of lymphatics.

Fat absorption

Studies of fat absorption *per se* are few.[35,58,59] In heterotopic canine ileal allograft recipients on conventional immunosuppression, the absorption of lauric acid mixed with bile salts was shown to increase from 10 per cent to 30 per cent of the amount administered over the early postoperative period before rejection caused a sharp decline.[24] Triglyceride absorption showed similar changes. Tritium-labelled oleic acid from canine orthotopic grafts in recipients treated with cyclosporin demonstrated high absorption by two weeks post-transplantation, which compared favourably with autografts.[9] Recipients undergoing rejection did not absorb significant amounts of fat at any stage.

The measurement of faecal fat and faecal α 1-antitrypsin excretion in rat orthotopic allotransplants immunosuppressed with cyclosporin demonstrated significant faecal fat loss at about two weeks with a return to normal at one month.[60] These animals were specifically fed long-chain triglycerides to preferentially identify active lymphatic drainage pathways as opposed to short- or medium-chain triglycerides which would be absorbed directly into the portal blood. By one month postoperatively 96 per cent[61,62] of the ingested fat was absorbed.

In the clinical setting cyclosporin is administered orally in a fatty vehicle. Under experimental conditions cyclosporin has been supplied in powder form and dissolved in olive oil. The study of cyclosporin absorption by transplanted bowel obviously reflects the ability of the graft to take up fat and can be accurately measured by radio-immunoassay.[63] Allotransplanted and even autotransplanted bowel shows considerable impairment of cyclosporin uptake compared to normal bowel. The transplanted bowel does function, however, as animals which have undergone a total small intestinal resection take up almost no cyclosporin at all.[36]

The absorption has been proven to be via the lymphatics by experimental drainage of thoracic duct fistulae. In such animals, the cyclosporin level within the lymphatic effluent is extremely high while the level within the peripheral blood barely increases above the baseline. Experiments in this animal model have also shown that preconditioning of the bowel with olive oil is efficacious in increasing cyclosporin absorption.[36] Rejection of the graft results in considerably reduced absorption – a situation which is improved by reversing the immunological damage.

Intestinal adaptation, growth and metabolism

An important feature of the transplanted small intestine will be its ability to adapt to nutritional demands in the longer term. It is unlikely that very large lengths of small intestine will be transplanted for immunological as well as practical reasons. Therefore it is hoped that functional adaptation will occur much as is seen in animals with a small residual short loop following extensive small bowel resection. Studies have shown that such grafts will provide for survival and growth in rats with short bowel syndrome.[64]

A complex study of function, metabolism and growth has been performed in rats.[33] Immunosuppressed recipients of either 40 cm allograft or isograft have been compared at 25 days. The recipients have all been shown to lose weight during the first 7 to 10 days. Thereafter, weight remains stable at about 20 per cent below the operative weight. In a careful comparison of 150 isografts in non-immunosuppressed animals at 150 days there appears to be an increase in villous height and crypt depth compared to intestine harvested from normal littermates. Interestingly, the absorption of 34 glucose is supra-normal in these recipients.

Following massive small bowel resection, the intestine is known to undergo hypertrophy, hyperplasia and dilatation.[65,66] The anatomical changes probably result in a functional compensation by slowing transit time, increasing the absorptive surface area and hence permitting normal nutrition and growth.

We do not know the mechanisms by which transplanted bowel adapts. It is reasonably certain that the extrinsic innervation does not play a major role. There are several possibilities which must include factors including gastrin, enteroglucagon and pancreatic enzymes, neural factors, and nutritional components.[67,68]

The mode of venous drainage of the graft is highly relevant from the point of view of immunosuppression. Drainage via the portal system is physiological. The impact of portal versus systemic drainage on isografts has been studied in rats over a time course of six months.[20] The liver weight of recipients has been very comparable between the portal and systemic drained recipients. This is in sharp contra-distinction to non-transplanted rats where a porto-caval shunt has been performed. In these animals there is liver atrophy over the six-month period.[69] Shunting is also accompanied by a deterioration in liver function[70,71] Serum ammonia levels are raised to approximately 140 mcg/ml in animals undergoing portocaval drainage of their grafts. This is considerably greater than the levels seen with portoportal anastomosis (84 mcg/ml) but does not compare with the much higher levels associated with portocaval shunting (560 mcg/ml). The serum triglyceride level in the transplanted animals was about 80 per cent of normal, but reduced to 50 per cent of normal in the presence of a portocaval shunt. Serum electro-phoresis for albumin and globulin remained normal.

Overall these experiments show that systemic drainage of transplanted bowel has a relatively minimal effect on the function of a normal liver. It is a matter of speculation, however, as to the effect of such changes on a liver already damaged by long-term parenteral nutrition.

Intestinal motility – normal

Intestinal movements are complex and do not merely involve aboral peristalsis of luminal content. Non-propulsive peristalsis, rhythmic segmentation of circular muscle, and pendular movements of longitudinal muscle all serve to provide a mixing function. The intestinal villi are also constantly alternating between contraction and relaxation and hence are exposed to varied luminal contents. Villus motility also promotes the movement of lymph along the central chylous vessels. Propulsive peristalsis consists of either short-segment activity affecting local chyme, or major movement, preceded by a phase of relaxation, which travels along the entire small bowel and can effectively sweep the lumen clean.

Intestinal motility is regulated primarily by the myenteric plexus. The external autonomic innervation appears to be of only secondary importance, as evidenced by the lack of change following vagotomy. The peristaltic events are elicited and maintained by stretching of the intestinal wall. Peristalsis is distinctly polarized and surgical reversal of a segment results in hold-up proximal to the operation. Villus movement is controlled by the submucosal plexus and to some extent by a locally produced hormone, villikinin.[72] Autonomic innervation has some influence over villus activity, the parasympathetic nerves causing contraction while the sympathetic fibres cause relaxation.

Experimental assessment

Experimental assessment of motility is best performed by placement of unipolar silver wire elec-

26. Donowitz M, Cusolito S, Battisti L, Fogel R, Sharp GW. Dopamine stimulation of active Na and Cl absorption in rabbit ileum. *J Clin Invest* 1982; **69,** 1008–16.
27. Sjovall H, Redfors S, Hallback DA, Eklund S, Jodal M, Lunsdren O. The effect of splanchnic nerve stimulation on blood flow distribution, villus tissue osmolarity and fluid and electrolyte transport in the small intestine of the cat. *Acta Physiol Scand* 1983; **117,** 359–65.
28. Brunnson I, Eklund S, Jodal M, Lundren O, Sjovell H. The effect of vasodilation and sympathetic nerve stimulation on net water absorption in the cat small intestine. *Acta Physiol Scand* 1979; **106,** 61–8.
29. Cheng EB, Bergenstai RM, Field M. Diarrhoea in streptozotocin-treated rats. Loss of adrenergic regulation of intestinal fluid and electrolyte transport. *J Clin Invest* 1985; **75,** 1666–70.
30. Quigley EMM, Thompson JS, Rose SG. The long-term function of canine jejuno-ileal-autotransplants. Insights into allograft physiology. *Transplant Proc* 1992; **24,** 1105–6.
31. Deltz E, Schroeder P, Gundlach M, Hansmann ML, Leimenstoll G. Successful clinical small bowel transplantation. *Transplant Proc* 1990; **22,** 2501.
32. Sigalet DL, Kneteman NM, Simpson I, Walker K, Thomson ABR. Intestinal permeability after small bowel transplantation and Cyclosporin treatment. *Transplant Proc* 1992; **24,** 1120–1.
33. Kirsch AJ, Kirsch SS, Kimura K, LaRosa CA, Jaffe BM. The adaptive ability of transplanted rat small intestine. *Surgery* 1991; **109,** 779–87.
34. Nordgren S, Cohen Z, MacKenzie R, Kinkelstein D, Greenberg GR, Langer B. Functional monitors of ejection in small intestinal transplants. *Am J Surg* 1984; **147,** 152–7.
35. Dennison AR, Collin J, Watkins RM, Millard PR, Morris PR. Segmental small intestinal allografts in the dog: 1. Morphological and functional indices of rejection. *Transplantation* 1987; **44,** 474–8.
36. Wassef R, Cohen Z, Nordgren S, Langer B. Cyclosporin absorption in intestinal transplantation. *Transplantation* 1985; **39,** 496–9.
37. Grant DR, Zhong R, Hurlbut D, Garcia B, Chen H, Lamont D, Wang P. Stiller C, Duff J. A comparison of heterotopic and orthotopic intestinal transplantation in rats. *Transplantation* 1991; **51,** 948–54.
38. Jenkins RT, Ramage JK, Jones DB, Collins SM, Goodacre RL, Hunt RH. Small bowel and colonic permeability to 51Cr-EDTA in patients with active inflammatory bowel disease. *Clin Invest Med* 1988; **11,** 151–5.
39. Teitelbaum DH, Dunaway DJ, Sonnino RE, Stellin G, Berend ME, Harmel RP. Leakage of intraluminal low molecular weight polyethylene glycol as a marker of small bowel transplant rejection. *J Paed Surg* 1989; **24,** 64–9.
40. Sladen GE, Dawson AM. An evaluation of perfusion techniques in the study of water electrolyte absorption in man: the problems of endogenous secretions. *Gut* 1968; **9,** 530–5.
41. Heinemann E, Meijssen MAC, deBruin RWF, Marquet RL, Molenaar JC. Electrophysiologic and histological monitoring of MHC matched and mismatched canine intestinal allografts. *J Paed Surg* 1991; **26,** 893–9.
42. Lee MD, Smith SD, Yunis EJ, Rowe MI. *In vivo* transmural potential difference: an early monitor of rejection in small bowel transplantation. *J Paed Surg* 1989; **24,** 767–70.
43. Meijssen MAC, Heineman E, deBruin RWF, Kate FJWT, Marquet RL, Molenaar JC. Detection of canine intestinal allograft rejection by *in vivo* electrophysiologic monitoring. *Transplantation* 1991; **51,** 955–9.
44. Madara JL, Kirkman RL. Structural and functional evolution of jejunal allograft rejection in rats and the ameliorating effects of Cyclosporin therapy. *J Clin Invest* 1985; **75,** 502–12.
45. Field M. Secretion of electrolytes and water by mammalian small intestine. In Johnson LR (ed.) *Physiology of the Gastrointestinal Tract*. New York, Raven Press, pp. 963–82, 1981.
46. Schultz SG. Ion coupled transport across biological membranes. In Andreoli TE, Hoffman JR, Fanestil DD (eds) *Physiology of Membrane Disorders*. New York, Plenum Press, pp. 925–62, 1978.
47. Lear PA, Watson AJM, Crane PW, Farthing MJG, Wood RFM. Autonomic function limits mucosal transport in Cyclosporin treated small intestinal transplants. *Transplant Proc* 1988; **20,** 436–42.
48. Crane PW, Clark C, Sowter C, Davies RL, Slavin G, Wood RFM, Lear PA. Cyclosporin toxicity in the small intestine. *Transplant Proc* 1990; **22,** 2432.
49. Ishii H, Hashimoto N, Kitada T, Kuroki T, Utsunomiya J. Analysis of malabsorption in small bowel transplants. *Transplant Proc* (Abstract), Second International Symposium on Small Bowel Transplantation, London, Ontario, 1991.
50. Schroeder P, Deltz E, Seifert J, Sandforth F, Thiede A. Absorptive capacity of the transplanted small bowel. *Gut* 1987; **2,** 275–9.
51. Hatcher PA, Deaton DH, Bollinger RR. Transplantation of the entire small bowel in inbred rats using Cyclosporin. *Transplantation* 1987; **43,** 478–84.
52. Diliz-Perez HS, McClure J, Bedetti C, Hong H-Q, de Santibanes E, Shaw BW, Van Thiel D, Iwatsuki S, Starzl TE. Successful small bowel allotransplantation in dogs with Cyclosporin and prednisolone. *Transplantation* 1984; **37,** 126–9.
53. Holmes HT, Yea SDJ, Winower SJ, Kawani N, Fortner JC. Absorption studies in canine jejunal allografts. *Ann Surg* 1971; **174,** 101–8.

54. Schroeder P, Gundlach M, Quaroni S, Hansmann ML, Schweizer E, Deltz E. Follow-up of small bowel transplantation by monoclonal antibodies against brush-border membranes. *Transplant Proc* 1990; **22,** 2476.
55. Kocandrle V, Houttuin E, Prohaska JV. Regeneration of the lymphatics after autotransplantation and homotransplantation of the entire small intestine. *Surg Gynaecol Obstet* 1966; **122,** 587–92.
56. Liu H, Teraoka S, Ota K, Nozawa M. Successful lymphangiographic investigation of mesenteric lymphatic regeneration after orthotopic intestinal transplantation in the rat. *Transplant Proc* 1992; **24,** 1113–14.
57. Schmid T, Korozsi G, Oberhuber G, Klima G, Margreiter R. Lymphatic regeneration after small bowel transplantation. *Transplant Proc* 1990; **22,** 2446.
58. Sigalet DL, Kneteman NM, Fedorak RN, Thomson ABR. Functional capacity of transplanted small bowel. *Transplant Proc* (Abstract), Second International Symposium on Small Bowel Transplantation, London, Ontario, 1991.
59. Stamford WP, Hardy MA. Fatty acid absorption in jejunal autograft and allograft. *Surgery* 1974; **75,** 496–502.
60. Kitigawa H, Ford EG, Sinatra F, Thomas D, Atkinson JB. Fecal fat, Cyclosporin, and a1-antitrypsin for assessment of small bowel function following transplantation. *J Paed Surg* 1991; **26,** 1091–6.
61. Senior JR. The place of medium chain triglycerides. *Am J Med Sci* 1969; **257** 1, 75–80.
62. Leyland FC, Fosbrooke AS, Lloyd JK. Use of medium chain triglyceride diets of children with malabsorption. *Arch Dis Child* 1969; **44,** 170–9.
63. Wolf BA, Daft MC, Koenig JW, Flye MW, Turk JW, Sloot MG. Measurement of Cyclosporin concentrations in whole blood HPLC and radioimmunoassay with a specific monoclonal antibody and ^{3}H- or^{125}-labelled ligand compared. *Clin Chem* 1989; **35,** 120–4.
64. Kimura K, Money SR, Jaffe BM. Short-segment orthotopic intestinal isografts and allografts in enterectomised rats. *Transplantation* 1978; **44,** 579–82.
65. Sonnino RE, Teitelbaum DH, Dunaway DJ, Harmel RP Jr. Small bowel transplantation: survival of rats with lethal short gut syndrome. *J Paed Surg* 1989; **24,** 956–62.
66. Hanson WR, Osborne JW, Sharp JG. Compensation by the residual intestine after intestinal resection in the rat. *Gastroenterology* 1977; **72,** 692–700.
67. Nylander G, Olerud S. Intestinal adaptation following extensive resection in the rat. *Acta Chir Scand* 1962; **123,** 51–6.
68. Williamson RCN, Chir M, Buchholtz TW, Malt RA. Humoral stimulation of cell proliferation in small bowel after transection and resection in rats. *Gastroenterology* 1978; **75,** 249–54.
69. Wittman T, Crenner F, Koenig M, Grenier M. Adaptive changes in postprandial motility after resection and bypass. *Dig Dis Sci* 1988; **33,** 1370–6.
70. Fischer B, Fischer ER, Lee S. Experimental evaluation of liver atrophy and portacaval shunt. *Surg Gynaecol Obstet* 1967; **125,** 1253–8.
71. Lauterburg BH, Sautter V, Preisig R, Bircher J. Hepatic functional deterioration after portacaval shunt in the rat. Effects of sulphobromophthalein transport maximum, indocyanic green clearance and galactose elimination capacity. *Gastroenterology* 1976; **71,** 221–7.
72. Kokas E, Johnston CC. Influence of refined villikinin on motility of intestinal villi. *Amer J Physiol* 1965; **208,** 1196–9.
73. Sarr MG, Kelly KA. Myoelectric activity of the autotransplanted canine jejuno-ilium. *Gastroenterology* 1981; **81,** 303–10.
74. Nemeth M, Harris MS, Ramaswamy K. Rat small intestine isografts have normal fasted and fed myoelectric activity and decreased absorption capacity. *Dig Dis Sci* 1987; **37,** 923–9.
75. DeWever I, Eeckhout C, Vantrappen G, Hellemans J. Disruptive effects of test meals on inter-digestive motor complex in dogs. *Am J Physiol* 1978; **235,** 661–5.
76. Code CF, Marlett JA. The interdigestive myoelectric complex of the stomach and small bowel of dogs. *J Physiol* 1975; **246,** 289–309.
77. Ormsbee HS III, Telford GL, Mason GR. Required neural involvement in control of canine migrating motor complex. *Am J Physiol* 1979; **237,** 451–6.
78. Weisbrodt NW, Copeland EM, Moore EP. Effect of vagotomy on electrical activity of the small intestine of the dog. *Am J Physiol* 1975; **228,** 650–4.
79. Aeberhardt PF, Magnenat LD, Zimmerman WA. Nervous control of migratory myoelectric complex of the small bowel. *Am J Physiol* 1980; **238,** 102–8.
80. Taguchi T, Zorychta E, Sonnino R, Guttman FM. Small intestine transplantation in the rat: effect of physiological properties of smooth muscle and nerves. *J Ped Surg* 1989; **24,** 1258–63.
81. Taguchi T, Zorychta E, Sonnino RE, Guttman FM. Function of smooth muscle and nerve after small intestinal transplantation in the rat: effect of storing donor bowel in Eurocollins. *J Ped Surg* 1989; **24,** 634–8.
82. Schiller WR, Suriyapa C, Mutchler JHW, Gohara JF, Anderson MC. Motility changes associated with canine intestinal allografting. *J Surg Res* 1973; **15,** 379–84.

4

Rejection and graft-versus-host disease

Richard F M Wood and Celia L Ingham Clark

Introduction

The small bowel is unique among solid organ grafts in having such a large lymphoid component. In addition to the organized structures of the Peyer's patches and lymph nodes, the lamina propria also contains a vast mass of mobile lymphocytes. There is a small additional population in the intraepithelial compartment where the lymphocytes lie on the basement membrane between the enterocytes of the villi. The size of the lymphocyte population is the reason that the small bowel is both a major target for rejection and an effective platform for the development of graft-versus-host disease (GVHD).

Rejection

Contact between graft and host antigens

In small bowel transplantation the immunological mechanism of rejection is essentially the same as in all other types of organ allografts. The initial trigger for the sensitization process is the contact between the Class I and Class II antigens expressed on the graft, particularly its lymphocyte population, and the lymphocytes of the recipient. The enterocytes strongly express HLA antigens but in the initial stages of rejection their contact with host lymphocytes is probably minimal. In other organ grafts the sensitization process largely occurs within the transplant itself by contact between infiltrating host cells and graft dendritic cells. In small bowel transplantation, due to the extensive donor cell migration from the graft, there is an additional potential for significant sensitization to take place within host lymphoid tissue.

The development of host sensitization

Two signals are required to trigger T lymphocyte proliferation: the presentation of the sensitizing antigen and a soluble mediator, interleukin-1 (IL-1). Macrophages play a pivotal role in this process secreting IL-1 and facilitating the contact between graft antigen and host cells. Foreign HLA antigens are recognized by the T cell receptor in association with host Class I and Class II antigens.[1] This is part of a developmental protective mechanism to prevent activation of the immune system by self-antigens. The identification of a foreign protein stimulates the synthetic machinery of the T cell to induce proliferation. Unless subverted by immunosuppression a population of CD4 positive lymphocytes will develop with the capacity to trigger the rejection process. These cells secrete the lymphokine interleukin-2 (IL-2) which is capable of sensitizing CD8 positive cells to become involved in the process. Together these cells home to the graft and cause an interstitial infiltrate. They have the potential to destroy graft cells by the secretion of cytotoxic factors. However, it is through the production of an additional range of lymphokines that they probably exert their maximal effects. The lymphokines, IL-1, IL-6 and TNF augment the inflammatory reaction within the graft by attracting other cells – such as polymorphs and macrophages – to take part in the destructive process. This is the classical process of cell-mediated immunity thought to be largely responsible for early acute rejection in all forms of organ allografts.[2] At the same time there is also the potential for antibody-mediated immunity to occur. Through cell-cell cooperation involving T cell help, B lymphocytes become sensitized to graft antigen and secrete antibody directed against graft tissue. This process was originally felt to be of minimal importance since it was difficult to detect significant levels of circulating antibodies directed against graft antigen, even during severe rejection episodes. However, following removal of an irreversibly rejected graft it was frequently possible to find high levels of circulating antibodies once they were deprived of a target tissue to bind to.[3] Antibodies involved in rejection appear to have a particular predilection to home to the endothelium of the graft with the potential to disrupt the micro-circulation.

Acute rejection in small bowel transplantation

Much of the evidence of the rejection process in small bowel transplantation comes from experiments conducted with inbred strains of rats. In transplants between two genetically distinct strains there is the potential for both rejection and GVHD. For example, between the DA and PVG strains which differ at the RT1 locus (DA – RT1a, PVG – RT1c) or the Lewis and Brown Norway, strains where there is an RT1c difference.[4] Alternatively, rejection can be studied as an isolated phenomenon in semi-allogeneic transplants where bowel from an F1 hybrid (the offspring of two different parental strains) is transplanted into an animal of one of the two parental strains;[5] for example, (PVG × DA) → DA or (Lewis × BN) → Lewis. Rejection is the dominant force following fully-allogeneic transplantation in the absence of immunosuppression. Transplantation from a BN donor to a Lewis recipient rat will result in destruction of the graft within 7 days without any overt evidence of GVHD. The time course of the rejection is identical in the semi-allogeneic (Lewis × BN) → Lewis model.[6] By day 2 after transplantation there is evidence of an increase in the size of the mesenteric lymph node of the gut (in the rat this is a single elongated structure in contrast to the multiple groups of distinct lymph nodes found in humans). The increase in node size is mainly due to an influx of host cells but may also be partly due to the lymphatic disruption associated with transplantation. By day 3 the Peyer's patches are also enlarged. Up until this point the mucosa of the graft appears histologically normal but from day 4 onwards the lymphocytic forces massing within the organized lymphoid tissues are released on the gut itself. There is an obvious increase in the numbers of cells within the lamina propria particularly around the base of the crypts. There is also perivascular cuffing of lymphocytes and it seems that the vascular endothelium is a primary target for attack. Radiological studies of perfusion-fixed specimens have shown that attenuation of the micro-circulation of transplanted small bowel precedes histological evidence of mucosal damage.[7] By day 5 there are clear signs of mucosal damage. There is evidence of crypt lengthening and blunting of the villi. The villus tips become oedematous. This change is the prelude to mucosal destruction with sloughing of villus tips progressing rapidly to complete mucosal destruction. The time-course to mucosal destruction depends on the strain combination used but it is usually complete by day 10.[6]

Rejection patterns in other animal species

In outbred dogs the majority of studies report similar histological changes to those described in the rat. In most non-immunosuppressed animals there is evidence of mucosal destruction within 7–10 days of transplantation.[8,9] Interestingly, there has been a report that histological changes equivalent to those occurring in rejection may be seen in the first few days after autotransplantation.[10] It is clear that ischaemia and reperfusion injury may cause villus damage, which may complicate the interpretation of biopsies in the early post-transplant period. Careful assessment of multiple biopsies from rejecting small bowel have shown that, in the initial stages, the rejection changes are patchy.[10,11]

In the pig model of small bowel transplantation there have been no detailed studies of acute rejection. However, untreated animals die at around 7–10 days with evidence of severe mucosal damage consistent with the end-stage rejection changes seen in other species.[12,13,14]

gresses,[37,38] but this does not precede histological evidence of rejection.[38,39] Also, as the mucosal barrier fails unlabelled glucose is lost into the intestine, and labelled glucose may be broken down by bacteria within the gut lumen. Therefore the test may become unreliable in advanced rejection.[40] Peristaltic activity is lost in rejecting small bowel grafts, but only after overt histological changes have taken place.[39] Myoelectrical activity persists despite mucosal breakdown.[41] Motility studies are of undoubted interest in small bowel transplant research but are likely to be of little practical value in detecting rejection.

Monocyte procoagulant activity (PCA) in the blood of small bowel transplant recipients is raised during acute rejection. PCA is a T lymphocyte-regulated response which gives a measure of the effector function of immunologically activated monocytes, macrophages, and vascular endothelial cells.[42] In a rat model peripheral blood PCA has been shown to rise before histological signs of rejection can be detected.[43] However, the rise in PCA is not specific to rejection, and can be induced by sepsis. Therefore although it has been used in clinical transplantation, the diagnosis of rejection must be corroborated by evidence from another test such as graft histology.[44]

In summary, monitoring of small bowel allografts in large animal models and in humans requires the use of several tests, usually including graft histology and immunohistology, and a functional test, in order to obtain an accurate assessment since most of the tests available are not specific. There is a need for a sensitive, specific method of detecting rejection, which preferably does not require repeated graft biopsy. Mobile graft cells can be detected in many host tissues – for example spleen, lymph nodes, and blood – following small bowel transplantation but disappear during acute rejection. This sudden loss of graft cells from host tissues might serve as a useful indicator of rejection particularly if a reliable system of peripheral blood monitoring can be established.[45]

Graft-versus-host disease

Graft-versus-host disease (GVHD) is a major problem in bone marrow transplantation although it is almost unknown in solid organ transplantation. The basic conditions necessary for the development of GVHD were established many years ago.[46] They include:

1. Mature immunocompetent cells in the graft.
2. Host histocompatibility antigens which are not present in the graft.
3. Little immunological reaction by the host towards the graft, at least for long enough to permit GVHD to develop.

The T cell component of a bone marrow graft is able to populate the organized lymphoid tissue of the recipient and then go on to infiltrate the liver and the skin stimulating immunological reactions characterized by the release of lymphokines, in particular TNFα[47] and γ Interferon.[48] The reaction is also associated with an increase in natural killer cell activity.[49] The NK cells are thought to be effector cells in the reaction, contributing to the non-specific damage as they do in rejection.[50] Skin changes in GVHD progress from a maculopapular rash to exfoliative dermatitis in the full-blown disease. In the liver peri-portal infiltration of lymphocytes results in cholestasis and jaundice. The gut is also a major target for attack and this leads to diarrhoea.[51] In rodent experiments two stages of graft-versus-host reaction can be identified. First there is a proliferative phase induced by helper T cells[52] and associated with non-specific cytotoxicity. This leads to an increase in the number of intraepithelial lymphocytes (IEL) and a raised crypt cell production rate (CCPR).[53,54] Crypt elongation parallels the increase in NK cell activity.[55] After approximately 3 days a second, destructive phase develops. The CCPR falls to zero and cytotoxic T cells can be detected in the lamina propria.[54] At this stage there is villous shortening and the host animals become clinically unwell. This destructive stage is believed to result from the continued local production of lymphokines.[55]

In small bowel transplantation it appears that rejection and graft-versus-host disease exist in a dynamic equilibrium. If rejection is totally suppressed, then the conditions are set for the graft lymphocytes to proliferate and cause GVHD. If host immune responses remain active, graft lymphocytes are held in check. GVHD has been intensively investigated in rat models. Using the reverse of the semi-allogeneic rejection model, that is transplantation from parental strain to F1 hybrid, GVHD occurs as an isolated phenomenon.[5] In the absence of immunosuppression overt GVHD will develop by around 10 to 15 days after transplantation in most semi-allogeneic combinations. The animals adopt a hunched posture with marked erythema of the paws and ears. They lose weight and develop diarrhoea. Most die of systemic sepsis following bacterial translocation from the gut.[30] Few animals survive beyond 21 days. The immunological reaction appears to be particularly intense within the spleen. There is marked splenic enlargement and the 'relative splenic weight' is used as a measure of the severity of GVHD ('relative splenic weight' is the weight of the spleen in the transplanted animal as a proportion of its total body weight at the time of death).[56] The graft cells which infiltrate the spleen demonstrate specific anti-host cytotoxicity when isolated and tested *in vitro* against recipient strain lymphocytes.[57]

Graft cell migration to the host

As indicated earlier in this chapter, transplantation between two genetically distinct rat strains tends to result in rejection without the development of overt GVHD. However, experiments using strain-specific monoclonal antibodies have shown that, despite the absence of GVHD, there is still a major migration of graft cells to the host tissues.

Using the OX27 and MN4 monoclonal antibodies the migration patterns of graft lymphocytes to the host tissues have been studied. As indicated above in transplants from DA → PVG and PVG → DA there is rapid rejection of the graft with mucosal destruction by day 10 after transplantation. In these two models, if the host tissues are sampled on a daily basis, it is evident that despite the predominance of the rejection process there is a substantial migration of graft lymphocytes to certain host tissues. Sections of the Peyer's patches of the native bowel taken on day 1 after transplantation show a scattering of graft cells in the T cell areas (Fig. 4.2). There are similar numbers of cells in the mesenteric lymph node. Numbers of cells increase progressively until day 3–4 (Fig. 4.3). Thereafter there is a progressive reduction in cell numbers and by day 7 virtually all trace of graft cells has disappeared. Investigation of other host tissues shows a similar pattern of cell migration in the spleen, where the graft cells are concentrated around the periarteriolar lymphatic sheath. Small numbers of graft cells can also be detected in peripheral lymph nodes for the first 5–6 days after transplantation. We have been unable to identify any graft cells in the liver or the thymus. The migration of cells from the graft to the host is more marked in the PVG → DA than in the DA → PVG combination.[21] The pattern of graft cell migration to host tissues in non-immunosuppressed transplants in the PVG → DA combination is illustrated in Fig. 4.4. Transplantation from parent to F1 hybrid (the isolated GVHD model) leads to more aggressive GVHD in the PVG → PVG × DA

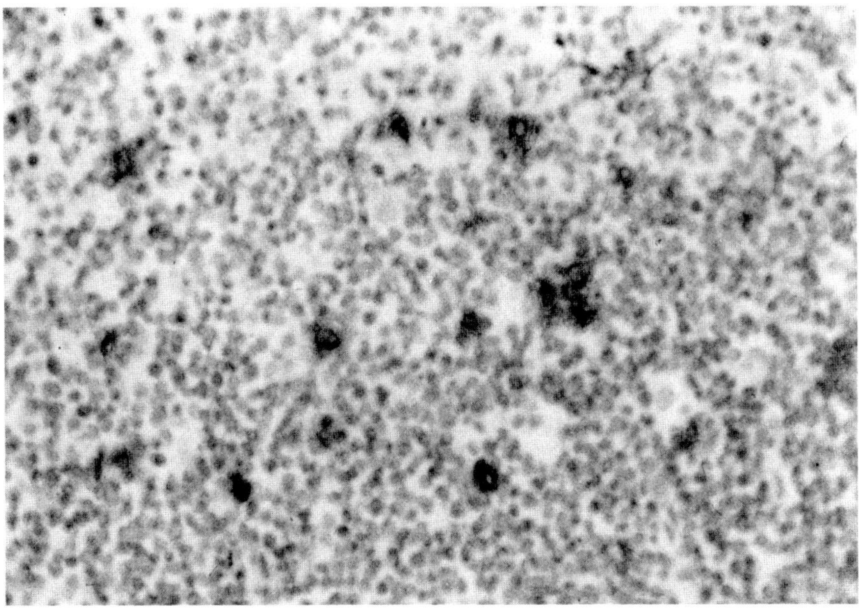

Fig. 4.2 Graft cell (PVG) infiltration of a Peyer's patch of host (DA) intestine 24 hours after transplantation. There is a scattering of graft lymphocytes, identified by the OX-27 monoclonal antibody using immunoperoxidase staining.

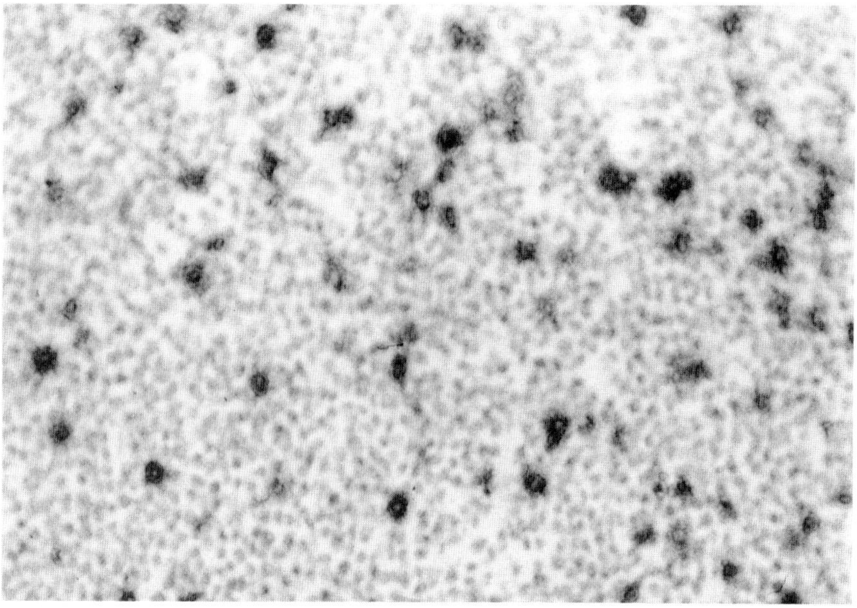

Fig. 4.3 More intensive infiltration of the host (DA) Peyer's patch by graft (PVG) cells 4 days after transplantation. In the non-immunosuppressed recipient the numbers of graft cells decline rapidly thereafter due to the host cytolytic response and loss of the lymphocyte source by destruction of the graft.

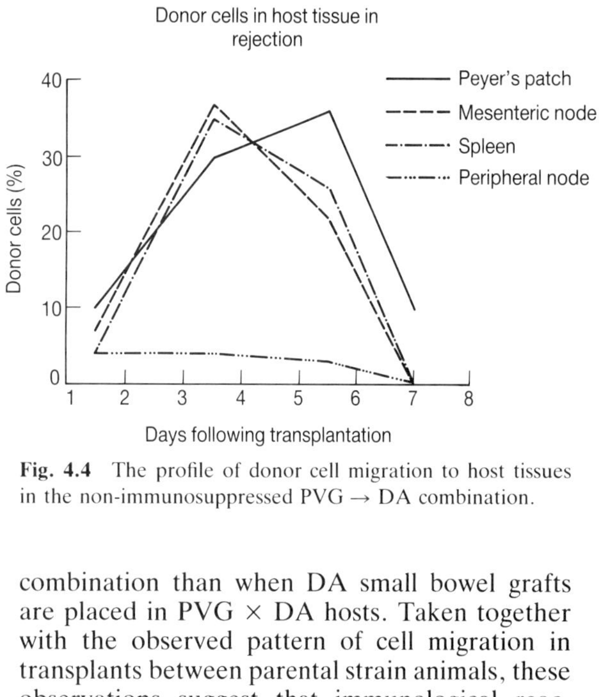

Fig. 4.4 The profile of donor cell migration to host tissues in the non-immunosuppressed PVG → DA combination.

combination than when DA small bowel grafts are placed in PVG × DA hosts. Taken together with the observed pattern of cell migration in transplants between parental strain animals, these observations suggest that immunological reactivity from PVG towards DA may be stronger than in the reverse direction. The larger cell migration from PVG donors to DA recipients may be a manifestation of a stronger GVH response.

In the absence of immunosuppression host immune responses overpower the infiltrating graft lymphocytes and since the source of replenishment is destroyed by rejection it is inevitable that the migration is transitory. When rejection is prevented by the use of continuous cyclosporin immunosuppression, a more intense and prolonged migration of graft cells is observed. In the PVG → DA combination at 7 days after transplantation 47 per cent of cells in the peri-arteriolar lymphatic sheath of the spleen (Fig. 4.5) and 60 per cent of the cells in the host mesenteric lymph nodes are of donor origin.[58] In long-term experiments fewer graft cells can be detected in host tissues; at day 56 approximately 8 per cent of the cells in the spleen and 14 per cent of the cells in the host mesenteric nodes remain of donor origin (Fig. 4.6).[24]

Occurrence of graft-versus-host disease in animal models

As already described the parent → F1 transplant combination always gives rise to GVHD. In outbred large animal models, clinical and pathological evidence of GVHD following small bowel transplantation has been more limited. In some series dogs with small bowel allografts have died between 10 and 30 days after transplantation with no evidence of rejection on graft histology, and it has been suggested that GVHD may have been present.[59,60] Histological changes consistent with

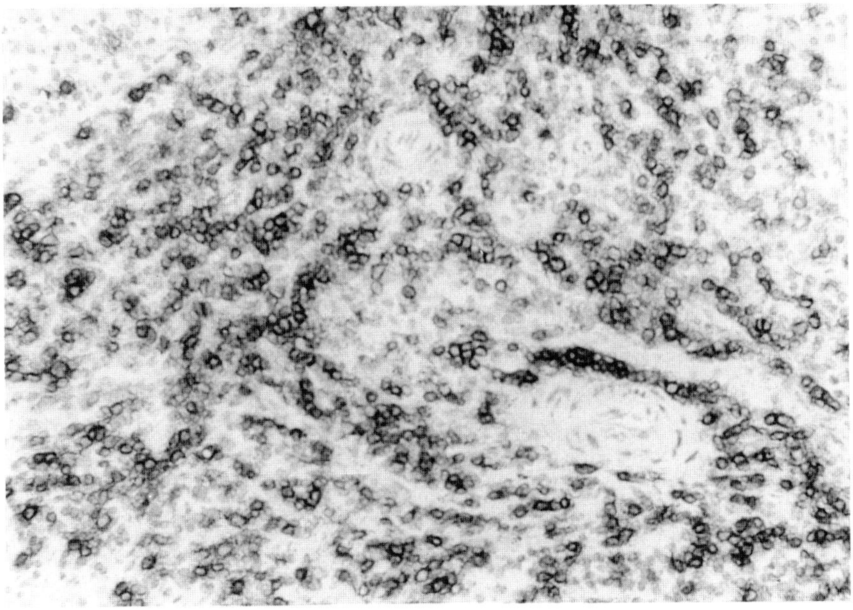

Fig. 4.5 Intensive graft cell infiltration of the peri-arteriolar lymphatic sheath of the host spleen 7 days after transplantation in a cyclosporin treated animal (PVG → DA).

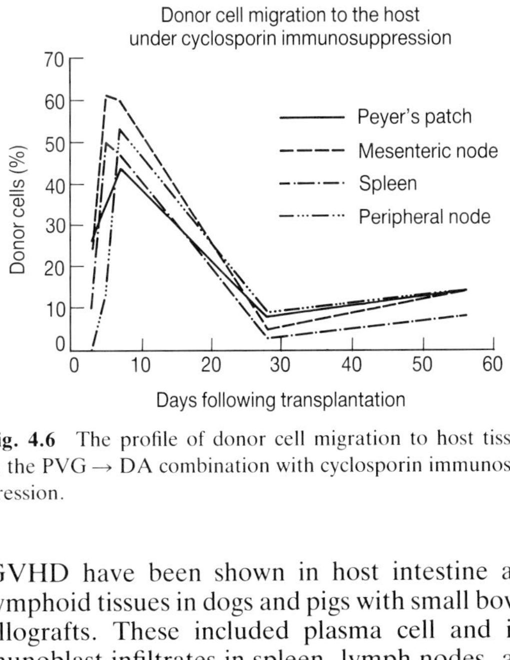

Fig. 4.6 The profile of donor cell migration to host tissues in the PVG → DA combination with cyclosporin immunosuppression.

GVHD have been shown in host intestine and lymphoid tissues in dogs and pigs with small bowel allografts. These included plasma cell and immunoblast infiltrates in spleen, lymph nodes, and gut.[61,62,14] However, no cutaneous GVHD has been found on clinical or histological assessment.[61,63]

Diagnosis of graft-versus-host disease

The clinical signs of GVHD are different from rejection. In humans, the diagnosis can be confirmed on the basis of skin or liver biopsy. The process also affects the large bowel and it has been suggested that there are diagnostic appearances on rectal biopsy.[64]

In experimental rat models, GVHD can be diagnosed by measuring relative splenic weight. In some fully-allogeneic strain combinations (e.g. BN → Lewis and WAG → BN), transient GVHD occurs if a short course of cyclosporin is given.[65,66] The other diagnostic test for GVHD in the rat is the Popliteal Lymph Node Assay. This test involves making a cell suspension from the recipient's spleen, injecting it into the footpad of another rat of the same strain as the recipient, then later harvesting the popliteal lymph nodes from that limb and from the contralateral limb. If the test is positive the lymph node from the limb which received the injection is enlarged compared with that of the contralateral limb.[74] Although this test has been shown to be valid in small bowel transplantation, it is rarely used as it involves the use of more experimental animals and alternative diagnostic tests are available.

Prevention of graft-versus-host disease

In bone marrow transplantation, established GVHD can sometimes be reversed using boluses of prednisolone, either with or without other immunosuppressants.[51] However, any episode of acute GVHD increases the likelihood of later development of chronic GVHD, therefore it is better to prevent GVHD when possible.

Again using bone marrow transplantation as the model, the risk of GVHD is related to the degree of antigenic disparity between donor and recipient, the number of lymphocytes transplanted (particularly T cells), the presence of bacterial infection,[51] and the age of the recipient.

T lymphocytes are essential for GVHD to occur in small bowel transplantation.[6] The effect of varying the number of lymphocytes included in a small bowel graft has been tested by transplanting short or long segments of small bowel. Varying the length of the graft does not affect the incidence of GVHD, but does affect its severity. Shorter grafts are associated with better survival following the development of GVHD.[67,68] In certain strain combinations GVHD has been completely abrogated by removing the graft mesenteric lymph node prior to transplantation.[57,69] This effect may be due to the large reduction in the lymphocyte content of the graft which this produces. However, in the PVG → DAX combination, excision of the mesenteric node only prolongs graft survival by a few days.[58]

Reducing graft lymphocytes

Irradiation of the donor or of the small bowel graft can prevent GVHD. Donor irradiation (700 or 950 rad) was effective in rats,[5,57] but would be impractical in the clinical setting. Graft irradiation has been used in dogs and in rats. In dogs, although the end-point of diagnosis was less clear, GVHD was apparently prevented by low-dose graft irradiation (50 rad), whereas high-dose irradiation (150 rad) brought about early graft necrosis.[60] In rats up to 500 rad was ineffective, and only a dose of 1000 rad could prevent the development of GVHD.[70] By 6 months after transplantation there was no evidence of radiation damage to the bowel on histological or functional testing. In human transplantation a radiation dose which would prevent GVHD without causing damage to the bowel has not been established. If the graft is irradiated *ex vivo* it may tolerate higher radiation doses because it is ischaemic.[71]

Donor pretreatment with antilymphocyte serum or globulin has also been used to prevent GVHD caused by small bowel transplants (see Chapter 9). It appears to work well when given from 48 hours before transplantation, but is not effective when given in the immediate peritransplant period.[72] The need for donor pretreatment would limit its usefulness in clinical transplantation.

In bone marrow transplantation other means of reducing graft lymphocytes have been employed. These include the use of specific anti-T cell monoclonal antibodies either alone or linked to magnetic beads so that physical separation of the T lymphocytes from the rest of the graft may be effected. More recently anti-T cell monoclonal antibodies have been linked to toxic agents such as ricin in order to produce specific T cell immunotoxins. Such agents have been successful in reducing the incidence of GVHD following bone marrow transplantation. In small bowel transplantation similar conjugates in a rat model prolonged survival but did not prevent the eventual development of fatal GVHD.[73,74]

Increasing immunosuppression

Cyclosporin has some effect on GVH reactivity *in vitro*,[75] but has been less effective in clinical bone marrow transplantation.[51] It does not appear to have entirely prevented GVHD in clinical intestinal transplantation. In semi-allogeneic experimental rat models a short course of CsA can prevent small bowel rejection, but continuous treatment is required to forestall GVHD.[6] CsA reduces anti-host GVH reactivity, but does not completely abolish it.[57] In large animal models continuous CsA treatment does not completely prevent GVHD.[14]

Recently the effects of CsA and FK 506 have been compared. In bone marrow transplantation FK 506 appears to be more effective than CsA in preventing GVHD.[76] Similar results were obtained in small bowel transplantation, where a short course of FK 506 seemed to provide extended protection against GVHD.[17]

Graft-versus-host reactions in human small bowel transplantation

In human transplantation donor cells have been detected in the recipient's peripheral blood.[33,77] In some cases this has been associated with overt GVHD. In Grant's first successful small bowel transplant, transient GVHD was observed. The patient developed a characteristic skin rash and biopsy confirmed the diagnosis.

Conclusion

There is evidence that a balance exists between the opposing immunological forces of rejection and GVHD. Measures which significantly reduce the risk of rejection appear to increase the incidence of GVHD. It appears that a substantial episode of rejection may obviate the risk of GVHD. In cell migration studies in rats, postponing the administration of cyclosporin immunosuppression until the third day after transplantation led to almost complete abrogation of graft cell migration to the host while still preventing irreversible rejection from developing.[45] In human small bowel transplants, the patients who have developed overt signs of GVHD have done so *before* they have undergone any rejection episode. When acute rejection takes place donor cells disappear from host tissues. Therefore the high incidence of acute rejection in small bowel transplants may be the reason for the paucity of reported instances of GVHD. More sophisticated measures to prevent rejection may increase the risk of GVHD.

Summary

1. The small bowel is highly immunogenic and provides a potent stimulus for the development of rejection. At the same time the large lymphoid component of the graft provides a source of cells capable of causing GVHD.
2. There are substantial exchange migrations of lymphocytes between host and graft. The replacement of graft lymphocytes by recipient cells does not necessarily indicate rejection.
3. The diagnosis of rejection requires functional as well as histological tests.
4. Effectively suppressing rejection may increase the risk of GVHD. There may therefore be logic in pursuing methods of reducing graft immunogenicity, which may reduce the risks of both rejection and GVHD, rather than simply increasing host immunosuppression.

References

1. Tilney NL, Kupiec-Weglinski JW, Heidecke CD, Lear PA, Strom TB. Mechanisms of rejection and prolongation of vascularised organ allografts. *Immunol Rev* 1984; **77,** 185–216.
2. Wagner H, Feldmann M, Boyle W, Schrader JW. Cell-mediated immune response *in vitro*. *J Exp Med* 1972; **136,** 331–43.
3. Wood RFM. Monitoring after transplantation. In Morris PJ (ed.) *Kidney Transplantation, Principles and Practice*, 2nd edn. London, Grune & Stratton, pp. 388–91, 1984.
4. Gill TJ III, Kunz HW, Misra DN, Cortese Hassett AL. The major histocompatibility complex of the rat. *Transplantation* 1987; **43,** 773–85.
5. Monchik GJ, Russell PS. Transplantation of small bowel in the rat: technical and immunological considerations. *Surgery* 1971; **70,** 693–702.
6. Kirkman RL, Lear PA, Madara JL, Tilney NL. Small intestine transplantation in the rat – Immunology and function. *Surgery* 1984; **96,** 280–6.
7. Crane PW, Ingham Clark CL, Sowter C, Davies RL, Slavin G, Wood RFM et al. Microvascular changes induced by cyclosporine. *Transplant Proc* 1991; **23,** 487.
8. Holmes JT, Klein MS, Winawer SJ, Fortner JG. Morphological studies of rejection in canine jejunal allografts. *Gastroenterology* 1971; **61,** 693–706.
9. Cohen Z, Nordgren S, Lossing A, Cullen J, Craddock G, Langer B. Morphological studies of intestinal allograft rejection. *Dis Colon Rectum* 1984; **27,** 228–34.
10. Millard PR, Dennison A, Hughes DA, Collin J, Morris PJ. Morphology of intestinal allograft rejection and the inadequacy of mucosal biopsies in its recognition. *Br J Exp Pathol* 1986; **67,** 687–98.
11. Schmid T, Oberhuber G, Korozsi G, Kuma G, Margreiter R. Histological pattern of small bowel allograft rejection in the rat. Mucosal biopsies do not provide sufficient information. *Gastroenterology* 1989; **96,** 1529–32.
12. Ricour C, Revillon Y, Arnaud-Battandier F, Ghnassia D, Weyne P, Lauffenburger A, et al. Successful small bowel allografts in piglets using cyclosporin. *Transplant Proc* 1983; **15,** 3019–26.
13. Grant D, Duff J, Zhong R, Garcia B, Lipohar C, Keown P, et al. Successful intestinal transplantation in pigs treated with cyclosporine. *Transplantation* 1988; **45,** 279–84.
14. Kaneko H, Hancock W, Schweizer RT. Progress in experimental porcine small bowel transplantation. *Arch Surg* 1989; **124,** 587–92.
15. Wassef R, Cohen Z, Nordgren S, Langer B. Cyclosporin absorption in intestinal transplantation. *Transplantation* 1985; **39,** 496–9.
16. Lee KKW, Schraut WH. Structure and function of orthotopic small bowel allografts in rats treated with cyclosporine. *Amer J Surg* 1986; **151,** 55–60.
17. Hoffman AL, Makowka L, Banner B, Cai X, Cramer DV, Pascualone A, et al. The use of FK 506 for small intestine allotransplantation. *Transplantation* 1990; **49,** 483–90.
18. von Willebrand E, Taskinen E, Ahonen J, Häyry P. Recent modifications in fine needle aspir-

ation biopsy of human renal allografts. *Transplant Proc* 1983; **15,** 1195–7.
19. Milton AD, Fabre JW. Massive induction of donor-type class I and class II MHC antigens in rejecting cardiac allografts in the rat. *J Exp Med* 1985; **161,** 98–112.
20. Jefferies WA, Green JR, Williams AF. Authentic T helper CD4 (W3/25) antigen on rat peritoneal macrophages. *J Exp Med* 1985; **162,** 117–27.
21. Lear PA, Cunningham AJ, Crane PW, Wood RFM. Lymphocyte migration patterns in small bowel transplants. *Transplant Proc* 1989; **21,** 2881–2.
22. Ingham Clark CL, Cunningham AJ, Crane PW, Wood RFM, Lear PA. Lymphocyte infiltration patterns in rat small-bowel transplants. *Transplant Proc* 1990; **22,** 2460.
23. Hell K, Gundlach M, Schmidt P, Hansmann M-L, Schroeder P, Deltz E. Immunohistochemical analysis of immunocompetent cells involved in small-bowel rejection in the rat. *Transplant Proc* 1990; **22,** 2461–2.
24. Ingham Clark CL, Lear PA, Wood S, Lennard-Jones JE, Wood RFM. Potential candidates for small bowel transplantation. *Br J Surg* 1992; **79,** 424–6.
25. Grover R, Ingham Clark CL, Pockley AG, Wood RFM, Lear PA. Host cell infiltration of graft tissues in a non-rejecting model of small bowel transplantation. *Br J Surg* 1992; **79,** 451.
26. Arnaud-Battandier F, Salmon H, Vaiman M, Revillon Y, Gallix P, Olivier M, et al. Small intestinal transplantation in swine with cyclosporine treatment: studies of the intestinal lymphoid populations. *Transplant Proc* 1985; **17,** 1440–1.
27. Murase N, Demetris AJ, Kim DG, Todo S, Fung JJ, Starzl TE. Rejection of multi-visceral allografts in rats: a sequential analysis with comparison to isolated orthotopic small bowel and liver grafts. *Surgery* 1990; **108,** 880–9.
28. Jalkanen S, Reichert RA, Gallatin WM, Bargatze RF, Weissman IL, Butcher EC. Homing receptors and the control of lymphocyte migration. *Immunol Rev* 1986; **91,** 39–60.
29. Grant D, Hurlbut D, Zhong R, Wang P, Chen H, Garcia B, et al. Intestinal permeability and bacterial translocation following small bowel transplantation in the rat. *Transplantation* 1991; **52,** 221–4.
30. Price BA, Cumberland NS, Ingham Clark CL, Wood RFM, Lear PA. Bacterial supercolonisation and the potential for translocation following small bowel transplantation. *Br J Surg* 1991; **78,** 1507.
31. Schroeder P, Schweizer E, Hansmann ML, Hell K, Gundlach M, Gassel J, et al. Monitoring in small bowel transplantation using cytochemistry and immunochemistry: a comparison of different techniques. *Transplant Proc* 1991; **23,** 675–6.
32. Garcia B, Zhong R, Wijsman J, Wang P, Chen H, Sutherland F, et al. Pathological changes following intestinal transplantation in the rat. *Transplant Proc* 1990; **22,** 2469–70.
33. Schroeder P, Sandforth F, Gundlach M, Deltz E, Thiede A. Functional adaptation of small intestinal mucosa after syngeneic and allogeneic orthotopic small bowel transplantation. *Transplant Proc* 1989; **21,** 2887–9.
34. Grant D, Lamont D, Zhong R, Garcia B, Wang P, Stiller C, et al. ^{51}Cr-EDTA: a marker for early intestinal rejection in the rat. *J Surg Res* 1989; **46,** 507–14.
35. Grant D, Wall W, Mimeault R, Zhong R, Ghent C, Garcia B, et al. Successful small bowel/liver transplantation. *Lancet* 1990; **335,** 181–4.
36. Madara JL, Kirkman RL. Structural and functional evolution of jejunal allograft rejection in rats and the ameliorating effects of cyclosporin therapy. *J Clin Invest* 1985; **75,** 502–12.
37. Cohen WB, Hardy MA, Quint J, State D. Absorptive function in canine jejunal autografts and allografts. *Surgery* 1969; **65,** 440–6.
38. Dennison AR, Collin J, Watkins R, Millard P, Morris PJ. Segmental small intestinal allografts in the dog. I Morphological and functional indices of rejection. *Transplantation* 1987; **44,** 474–8.
39. Hatcher PA, Deaton DH, Bollinger RR. Transplantation of the entire small bowel in inbred rats using cyclosporine. *Transplantation* 1987; **43,** 478–84.
40. Holmes JT, Yeh SD, Winawer SJ, Kawano N, Fortner JG. Absorption studies in canine jejunal allografts. *Ann Surg* 1971; **174,** 101–8.
41. Schiller WR, Suriyapa C, Mutchler JHW, Gohara SF, Anderson MC. Motility changes associated with canine intestinal allografting. *J Surg Res* 1973; **15,** 379–84.
42. Cole E, Cardella CJ, Schulman J, Levy G. Monocyte procoagulant activity and plasminogen activator: role in human renal allograft rejection. *Transplantation* 1985; **40,** 363–71.
43. Silverman R, Cohen Z, Levy G, Craig M, Cullen J, Langer B. Immune responses in small intestinal transplantation in the rat: correlation of histopathology and monocyte procoagulant activity. *Surgery* 1987; **103,** 395–402.
44. Cohen Z, Silverman RE, Wassef R, Levy GA, Burnstein M, Cullen J, et al. Small intestinal transplantation using cyclosporine. *Transplantation* 1986; **42,** 613–21.
45. Ingham Clark CL, Crane PW, Cunningham AJ, Wood RFM, Lear PA. An immunosuppressive regimen which reduces graft cell emigration following small bowel transplantation. *Transplant Proc* 1992; **24,** 1130.
46. Elkins WL, Guttman RD. Pathogenesis of a local graft-versus-host reaction: immunogenicity of

circulating leucocytes. *Science* 1968; **159,** 1250–1.
47. Piguet PF, Grau GE, Allet B, Vassalli P. TNF/cachectin is an effector of skin and gut lesions of the acute phase of graft-versus-host disease. *J Exp Med* 1987; **166,** 1280–9.
48. Guy-Grand D, Vassalli P. Gut injury in mouse graft-versus-host reaction: a study of its occurrence and mechanisms. *J Clin Invest* 1986; **77,** 1584–95.
49. Borland A, Mowat AMcI, Parrott DMV. Augmentation of intestinal and peripheral NK cell activity during the graft-versus-host reaction in mice. *Transplantation* 1983; **36,** 513–19.
50. Nemlander A, Saksela A, Häyry P. Are 'natural killer' cells involved in allograft rejection? *Eur J Immunol* 1983; **13,** 348–50.
51. Barrett AJ. Graft-versus-host disease: a review. *J Roy Soc Med* 1987; **80,** 368–73.
52. Mowat AMcI, Borland I, Parrott DMV. Hypersensitivity reactions in the small intestine. VII Induction of the intestinal phase of murine graft-versus-host reactivity by Lyt 2-T cells activated by I-A antigens. *Transplantation* 1986; **41,** 192–8.
53. Mowat AMcI, Ferguson A. Hypersensitivity reactions in the small intestine. VI Pathogenesis of the graft-*versus*-host reaction in the small intestinal mucosa of the mouse. *Transplantation* 1981; **32,** 238–43.
54. Mowat AMcI, Ferguson A. Intra-epithelial lymphocyte count and crypt hyperplasia measure the mucosal component of the graft-versus-host reaction in mouse small intestine. *Gastroenterology* 1982; **83,** 417–23.
55. Mowat AMcI, Felstein MV, Borland A, Parrott DMV. Experimental studies of immunologically mediated enteropathy: development of cell-mediated immunity and intestinal pathology during a graft-versus-host reaction in irradiated mice. *Gut* 1988; **29,** 949–56.
56. Pomposelli F, Maki T, Kiyoizumi T, Gaber L, Balogh K, Monaco AP. Induction of graft-versus-host disease by small intestinal allotransplantation in rats. *Transplantation* 1985; **40,** 343–7.
57. Deltz E, Ulrichs K, Schack T, Friedrichs B, Muller-Ruchholtz W, Muller-Hermelink HK. Graft-versus-host reaction in small bowel transplantation and possibilities for its circumvention. *Am J Surg* 1986; **151,** 379–86.
58. Ingham Clark CL, Price BA, Malcolm P, Lear PA, Wood RFM. Graft versus host disease in small bowel transplantation. *Br J Surg* 1991; **78,** 1007–9.
59. Lillehei RC, Idezuki Y, Feemster J, Dietzman RH, Kelly W, Merkel FK, et al. Transplantation of the stomach, intestine and pancreas: experimental and clinical observations. *Surgery* 1967; **62,** 721–41.
60. Cohen Z, MacGregor AB, Moore KTH, Falk RE, Langer B, Cullen JB. Canine small bowel transplantation: a study of the immunological responses. *Arch Surg* 1976; **111,** 248–53.
61. Williams JW, McClellan T, Peters TG, Nag S, Dean P, Banner B, et al. Effect of pre-transplant graft irradiation on canine intestinal transplantation. *Surg Gynecol Obstet* 1988; **167,** 197–204.
62. Fujiwara H, Grogan JB, Raju S. Total orthotopic small bowel transplantation with cyclosporine. *Transplantation* 1987; **44,** 469–74.
63. Reznick RK, Craddock GN, Langer B, Gilas T, Cullen JB. Structure and function of small bowel allografts in the dog: immunosuppression with cyclosporin A. *Can J Surg* 1982; **25,** 51–5.
64. Sale GE, McDonald GB, Shulman HM, Thomas ED. Gastrointestinal graft-versus-host disease in man: a clinicopathological study of the rectal biopsy. *Amer J Surg Pathol* 1979; **3,** 291–9.
65. Diflo T, Maki T, Balogh K, Monaco AP. Graft-versus-host disease in fully allogeneic small bowel transplantation in the rat. *Transplantation* 1989; **47,** 7–11.
66. Saat RE, Heineman E, De Bruin RWF, Marquet RL, Jeekel J. Total orthotopic allogeneic small bowel transplantation in rats. Attempts to ameliorate the graft-versus-host disease by irradiation and transfusions of the donor. *Transplantation* 1989; **47,** 451–3.
67. Deltz E, Muller-Hermelink HK, Ulrichs K, Thiede A, Muller-Ruchholtz W. Development of graft-versus-host reaction in various target organs after small intestinal transplantation. *Transplant Proc* 1981; **13,** 1215–16.
68. Kimura K, Money SR, Jaffe BM. The effects of size and site of origin of intestinal grafts on small bowel transplantation in the rat. *Surgery* 1987; **101,** 618–22.
69. Pirenne J, Lardinois F, D'Silva M, Fridman V, Boniver J, Mahieu P. Relevance of mesenteric lymph nodes to graft-versus-host disease following small bowel transplantation. *Transplantation* 1990; **50,** 711–14.
70. Lee KKW, Schraut WH. *In vitro* allograft irradiation prevents graft-versus-host disease in small bowel transplantation. *J Surg Res* 1985; **38,** 364–72.
71. Forsberg JO, Jung B, Larsson B. Mucosal protection during irradiation of exteriorised rat ileum. *Acta Radiol Oncol* 1978; **17,** 485–96.
72. Schaffer D, Maki T, Demichele SJ, Karlstad MD, Bistrian BR, Balogh K, et al. Prevention of graft-versus-host disease with preservation of allograft function by donor pre-treatment with anti-lymphocyte serum. *Transplantation* 1988; **45,** 262–9.
73. Smith GJ, Ingham Clark CL, Crane PW, Lear PA, Wood RFM, Fabre JW. *Ex vivo* perfusion of intestinal allografts with anti T cell monoclonal antibody/ricin A chain conjugates for the suppression

globulin, secretory IgA (sIgA), in intestinal secretions. In the last decade, mucosal immunity has been the subject of active research. It is now recognized that local mucosal immunity has important differences from systemic immunity, yet plays a major role in host defence.

The humoral component of the intestinal immune response is of special interest. Immunization of the intestine with antigen results in local sIgA secretion, not systemic IgG production. While the mechanisms by which this occurs are the subject of ongoing investigations and some controversy, a general outline of the process can be given. Macromolecular antigens are taken up by specialized cells called M cells located in Peyer's patches and delivered to antigen-presenting cells. Other antigens may be transported by intestinal absorptive epithelium and presented to the underlying CD4+ helper T cells in association with MHC class II molecules.[2–5] Either way, help is provided to responsive B cells, which differentiate and migrate to the mesenteric lymph nodes and enter the blood circulation via the thoracic duct. These B cells, primed in the intestine, circulate in the blood and return through 'homing' mechanisms to the lamina propria of the intestine or migrate to distant mucosal sites, where they mature into IgA synthesizing plasma cells.

IgA, synthesized in the lamina propria, can reach the intestinal lumen by two pathways. First, IgA is complexed with secretory component, transported across the epithelium, and secreted into the intestinal lumen. In the second pathway, IgA reaches the serum via mesenteric lymph vessels and the thoracic duct. Serum IgA is complexed with secretory component in hepatocytes and is actively and selectively transported through hepatocytes and secreted into bile and eventually the intestine.

The protective function of sIgA has been demonstrated in a variety of ways. sIgA can neutralize toxins, enzymes, and perhaps some viruses. sIgA also binds to surface molecules of bacteria and prevents bacterial adherence to intestinal epithelium and subsequent entrance to the portal blood circulation. sIgA is also thought to function as an opsonin for polymorphonuclear cells and macrophages. The significance of sIgA in protection has also been demonstrated by epidemiological studies. Infants who receive mother's milk containing large amounts of sIgA against intestinal pathogens have less disease produced by those organisms than infants receiving mother's milk without the antibodies or cow's milk.[6] Finally, the passive administration of a specific monoclonal sIgA can protect an experimental animal from mortality when challenged by a lethal dose of *Vibrio cholerae*.[7]

Viewed from another perspective, the clinical syndrome of selective or isolated IgA deficiency has been related to a number of abnormalities. Recurrent infections, primarily affecting the respiratory tract, but also affecting the gastrointestinal tract and other areas, are the most frequent manifestation associated with IgA deficiency. Of particular interest, autoantibodies and autoimmunity are often found in patients with IgA deficiency. In most cases these patients have autoantibodies with specificity for a variety of self-components as well as food proteins. In some cases the patients develop autoimmune diseases, including juvenile lupus erythematosus, type 1 diabetes mellitus, and various autoimmune endocrinopathies. A high frequency of allergic rhinitis and asthma has been noticed in IgA deficiency patients. Finally, a possible association of malignancy with IgA deficiency has been suggested.[8]

In addition to the unique humoral immune response mediated mainly by sIgA production, cell-mediated responses play an important role in intestinal mucosal immunity as well. In fact, small bowel contains the largest number of lymphocytes in the body; there are an estimated 10^{10} lymphocytes in a metre of human bowel, compared with 2.5×10^{10} in bone marrow, spleen and lymph nodes collectively.[9] The lymphocytes in the small bowel are divided into different compartments, with a characteristic phenotype and probably a different function. Intraepithelial T lymphocytes primarily express CD8, while those in the lamina propria express CD4. Characterization of the T cell receptor has shown that intraepithelial lymphocytes have a restricted repertoire compared to peripheral T cells.[10]

Functional studies have demonstrated that intestinal lymphocytes mediate most types of cytotoxicity. These include spontaneous or natural killer activity, lymphokine-activated killer cell activity, lectin-induced cytotoxicity and antibody-dependent cellular cytotoxicity (ADCC).[11–17] ADCC is particularly interesting as lymphocytes from the intestine require sIgA for ADCC, in contrast to splenic lymphocytes, which use IgG.

In addition to the humoral and cellular immune response in the local mucosal immune system, systemic antigen-specific unresponsiveness occurs concomitantly following intestinal immunization or feeding with a wide range of antigens.[18–19] This unresponsiveness, designated 'oral tolerance', is one of the important mechanisms to prevent hypersensitivity and autoimmunity to dietary antigens. Breakdown in 'oral tolerance' may result in immunological food hypersensitivity and autoimmunity as seen in some clinical enteropathies.[20] It is also possible that transplant surgeons may be able to take advantage of this phenomenon to generate systemic tolerance to transplanted organs through the intentional feeding of transplantation antigens.[21]

The production of sIgA by intestinal allografts

Since sIgA plays such an important role in the intestinal mucosal immune system, we elected to begin our investigation of the immune function of transplanted intestine with studies of sIgA production in transplanted small bowel. The aims of our studies were to determine: 1), if transplanted bowel made normal amounts of sIgA; 2), if the bowel could respond appropriately to a new immmunogen; 3), if the immune status of the donor or recipient altered the response; and 4) if the response was affected by immunosuppression.

For all of these studies we employed the same model, that of heterotopic, out of continuity small bowel transplantation in the rat. As the methods have been described elsewhere, they will be recapitulated here only in enough detail to make the subsequent experiments understandable.[22–30] Adult male Lewis × Brown Norway (LBN) F1 and Lewis (LEW) rats (Harlan Sprague Dawley, Indianapolis, IN), weighing 200–300 g, were used throughout. All transplants, both isografts and allografts, were carried out using a modification of the method of Monchik and Russell[31] previously described.[23] Ten centimetres of distal ileum were harvested as the graft; the donor aorta and portal vein were anastomosed end-to-side to the recipient aorta and vena cava respectively. The two ends of the graft were brought out as stomas to facilitate sample collection and immunization in some experiments. All allografts utilized LBNF1 rats as donors and LEW rats as recipients to avoid the possibility of graft-versus-host disease. In some experiments, Thiry–Vella loops created from 10 cm of distal ileum were used as controls.

Collection of samples for sIgA detection from grafts and loops was performed in a standard fashion. A catheter was inserted into one stoma, 2 ml of saline were flushed through the loop, and the effluent was collected from the other stoma. Air was instilled to be certain that as much of the flushing solution as possible was retrieved. The first sample was usually obtained prior to removal of the graft from the donor or at the time of creation of the Thiry–Vella loop. Subsequent samples were obtained through stomas at weekly intervals under ketamine anaesthesia. Samples generally contained some solid material which accumulated in the loop during the week between collections. The collected material was homogenized and centrifuged at 600 g for 10 minutes. Supernatants were collected and stored at −20°C until analysis for antibody.

All antibody determinations were made using ELISA assays developed in this laboratory and described in detail elsewhere.[23] The assays measured either total sIgA or specific sIgA directed against a given antigen. In the case of total sIgA, results are expressed as mg/ml of the intestinal samples, using a known bile standard as a control. For specific IgA against an administered antigen, results were expressed in arbitrary units, with one unit defined as that amount which gave an absorbance equal to a $1:10^5$ dilution of the bile standard. Data were analysed by analysis of variance for repeated measurements (ANOVA) following logarithmic transformation.

Total sIgA production

In our first experiment, we asked if transplanted bowel would make normal levels of sIgA without any deliberate immunization. As shown in Table 5.1, there were six groups, consisting of LBNF1 Thiry–Vella loops, LBNF1 isografts, and LBNF1-into-Lewis allografts, each with or without cyclo-

Table 5.1 Experimental groups for total sIgA

Group	CsA	n
1 LBNF1 loop	—	6
2 LBNF1 loop	day 0–7	6
3 LBNF1->LBNF1	—	6
4 LBNF1->LBNF1	day 0–7	5
5 LBNF1->Lewis	—	6
6 LBNF1->Lewis	day 0–7	6

sporin (CsA) immunosuppression. CsA (15 mg/kg/day) was administered by intramuscular injection for 7 days.

Samples were collected unless the grafts rejected, in which case collection became impossible. For untreated allografts, Group 5, this occurred after day 7 and prior to day 14 in all cases. Allografts in hosts treated with CsA were rejected after day 28; thus, this CsA regimen produced significant, but not indefinite, graft prolongation.

Total sIgA levels were not significantly different among all groups (Fig. 5.1). Whether compared over the entire course or at individual time points, statistical analysis failed to detect differences between isolated loops, isografts, or allografts. Cyclosporin had no effect on the total sIgA measured. Levels of sIgA were constant over time and significantly higher than preoperative (day 0) values, presumably as a result of accumulation of sIgA in isolated loops or grafts.

Response to immunization

In our second experiment, we asked if deliberate immunization would affect the levels of total sIgA production, and if the bowel would make a specific antibody response against the immunogen. Cholera toxin (CT) was selected as the immunogen for the experiments, as it is a well characterized intestinal antigen. Immunization was carried out by injection of 10 μg of CT (Calbiochem, LaJolla, CA) into the lumen of the bowel. Two doses, the initial dose and the booster dose, were given to each animal. The initial dose of CT was injected into the lumen of the graft during harvesting, while the booster dose was given by direct injection into the grafts 7 days after transplantation. The experimental groups are shown in Table 5.2.

Immunization with CT did not alter the pattern of secretion of total sIgA seen in the unimmunized animals (Fig. 5.2). Again, no differences over time or at individual points were identified among the experimental groups. Moreover, the measured levels were similar to those seen in the unimmunized animals.

In contrast, marked differences were detected among groups in the production of specific antibodies in response to immunization with CT (Fig. 5.3). Both Thiry–Vella loops (Group 1) and LBNF1 isografts (Group 2) promptly made specific sIgA anti-cholera toxin antibodies.

Immunosuppression with CsA delayed, but did not prevent, the specific sIgA production

Table 5.2 Experimental groups for cholera toxin immunization

Group	CsA	CT immunization	n
1 LBNF1 loop	—	day 0 and 7	10
2 LBNF1->LBNF1	—	day 0 and 7	9
3 LBNF1->LBNF1	day 0–7	day 0 and 7	10
4 LBNF1->Lewis	day 0–7	day 0 and 7	10

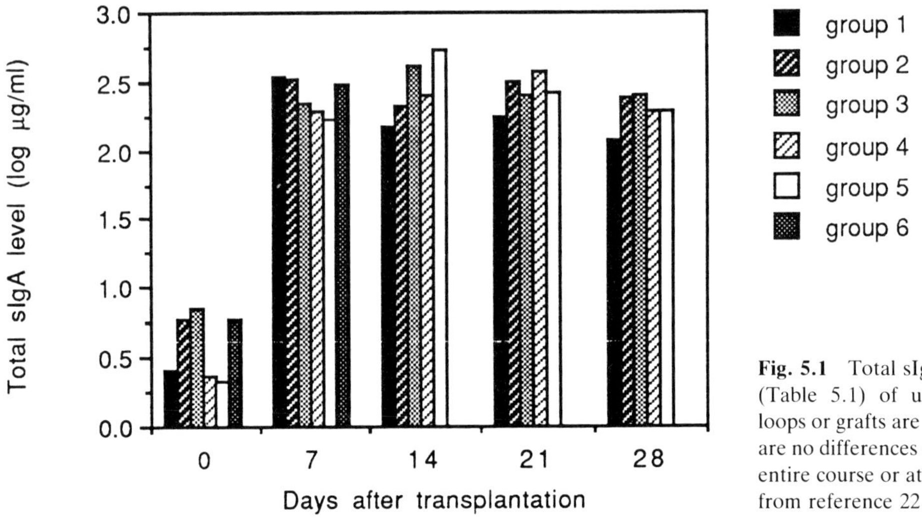

Fig. 5.1 Total sIgA levels in the six groups (Table 5.1) of unimmunized small bowel loops or grafts are shown as log μg/ml. There are no differences among the groups over the entire course or at any time point. (Modified from reference 22.)

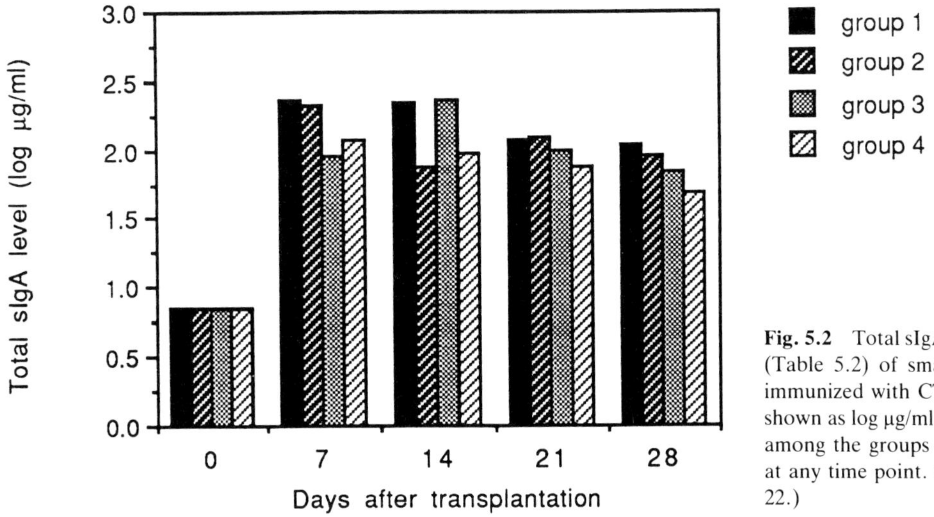

Fig. 5.2 Total sIgA levels in the four groups (Table 5.2) of small bowel loops or grafts immunized with CT. The total sIgA level is shown as log µg/ml. There are no differences among the groups over the entire course or at any time point. (Modified from reference 22.)

(Group 3). No detectable antibody was present at day 7, when CsA treatment ceased; thereafter, the antibody levels rose steadily and reached normal levels by day 21. Most importantly, allografts (Group 4) treated with CsA failed to make a significant anti-CT sIgA response. Overall production was different from each of the other three groups ($p < 0.05$).

Immune status of donor and recipient

The fact that transplanted small bowel made normal amounts of total sIgA, but failed to respond to a new specific antigen, suggested that the total sIgA produced might be in response to antigens previously seen by either the donor or the recipient. To test this hypothesis, and to determine if the immune status of donor or recipient would affect the response to a specific antigen, we performed a series of experiments in which either the donor or the recipient was primed with cholera toxin prior to transplantation.

In the first set of experiments, we asked if exposure of the donor to a specific antigen would result in transfer of the immune state. Four experimental groups were studied (Table 5.3). The small intestine of the donor was primed 7 days before transplantation by a direct injection of CT

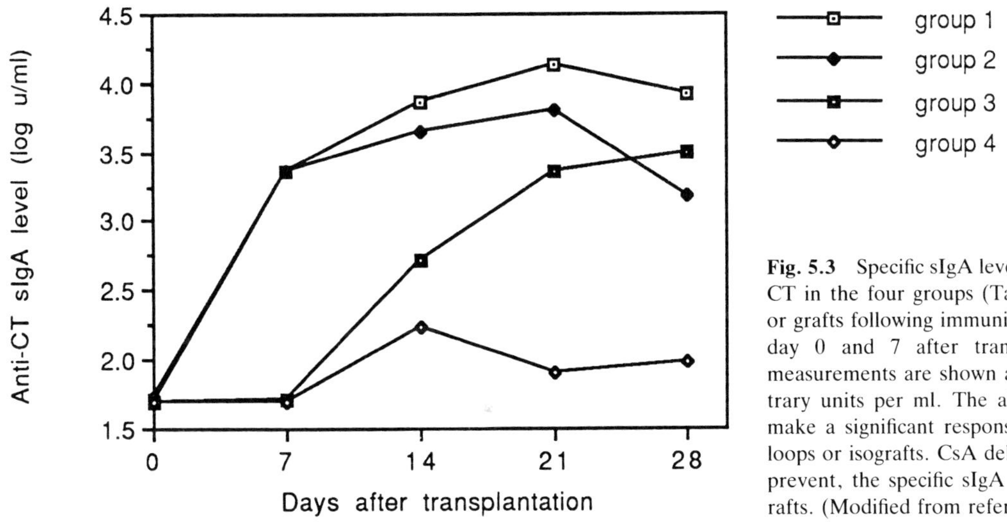

Fig. 5.3 Specific sIgA level directed against CT in the four groups (Table 5.2) of loops or grafts following immunization with CT at day 0 and 7 after transplantation. The measurements are shown as the log of arbitrary units per ml. The allografts failed to make a significant response compared with loops or isografts. CsA delayed, but did not prevent, the specific sIgA response in isografts. (Modified from reference 22.)

Table 5.3 Experimental groups with primed donor

Group	CsA	CT immunization	n
1 LBNF1 loop	—	day −7 and 7	9
2 LBNF1->LBNF1	—	day −7 and 7	9
3 LBNF1->LBNF1	day 0–7	day −7 and 7	9
4 LBNF1->Lewis	day 0–7	day −7 and 7	8

Table 5.4 Experimental groups with primed recipient CT immunization

Group	Day −7	Day 7	CsA	n
1 LBNF1–LBNF1	donor	graft	day 0–28	6
2 LBNF1–LBNF1	recipient	graft	day 0–28	7
3 LBNF1–Lewis	recipient	graft	day 0–28	7
4 LBNF1–Lewis	recipient	—	day 0–28	9

(10 μg) into the lumen of the intestine in four places. The second dose of CT was administered directly into the graft or loop on post-transplant day 7. Where indicated, CsA was given intramuscularly at dose of 20 mg/kg/d for 7 days.

Specific sIgA was detected at day 0 in all four donor-primed groups (Fig. 5.4). The levels of specific sIgA declined in all transplants, both isografts and allografts, at day 7, while levels in isolated Thiry–Vella loops increased ($p < 0.05$). This may represent technical factors, such as longer operation time or cold graft preservation, or it could be the result of lymphatic disruption in transplanted groups. However, the levels in transplanted groups rose after day 7 and no significant differences were detected among the four groups at day 14. Specific sIgA then fell significantly ($p < 0.05$) in allografts (Group 4) at days 21 and 28 as the grafts underwent gradual rejection.

In the next set of experiments, we primed the recipient rather than the donor before transplantation. From experiments described above, we know that naive donor-derived lymphocytes alone will be unable to make a specific sIgA response, at least if immunization takes place during CsA treatment. Therefore, if specific sIgA against CT can be detected in primed recipients, there must be a role for recipient-derived lymphocytes. Four groups were studied, as shown in Table 5.4. CsA was administered intramuscularly in each group for four weeks. Recipients were primed by direct injection into the bowel.

Naive intestinal grafts in primed recipients (Group 2–4) did not produce specific sIgA against CT on the day of transplantation, while grafts primed with CT 7 days before transplantation (Group 1) made significant levels of specific sIgA ($p < 0.05$) (Fig. 5.5). After CT boosting at day 7 post-transplantation, grafts in all boosted groups, both isografts (Group 1–2) and allografts (Group 3), made high titres of specific sIgA. There were no differences among these three groups at any time point after boosting ($p > 0.05$). Allografts in primed recipients without antigen restimulation (Group 4) failed to make significant specific sIgA

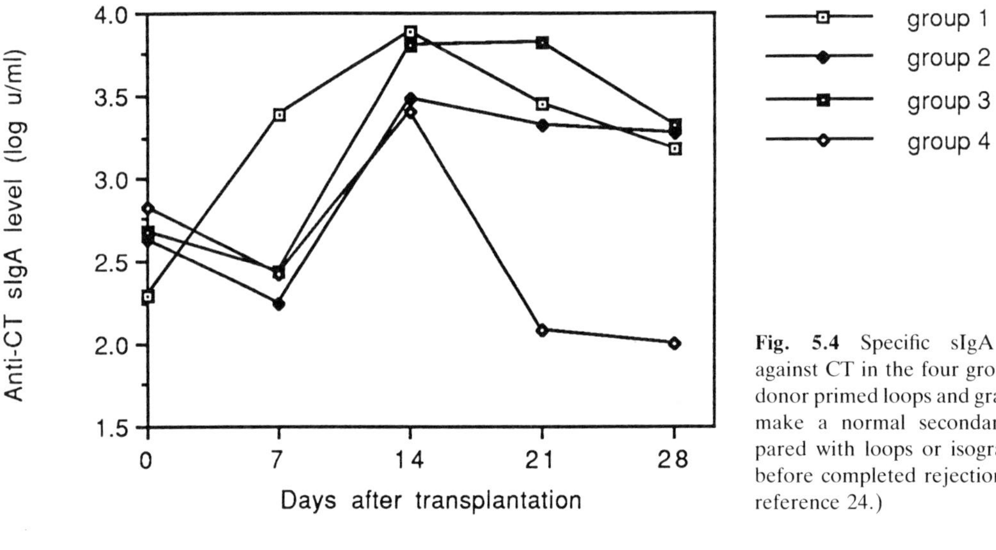

Fig. 5.4 Specific sIgA levels directed against CT in the four groups (Table 5.3) of donor primed loops and grafts. The allografts make a normal secondary response compared with loops or isografts until 2 weeks before completed rejection. (Modified from reference 24.)

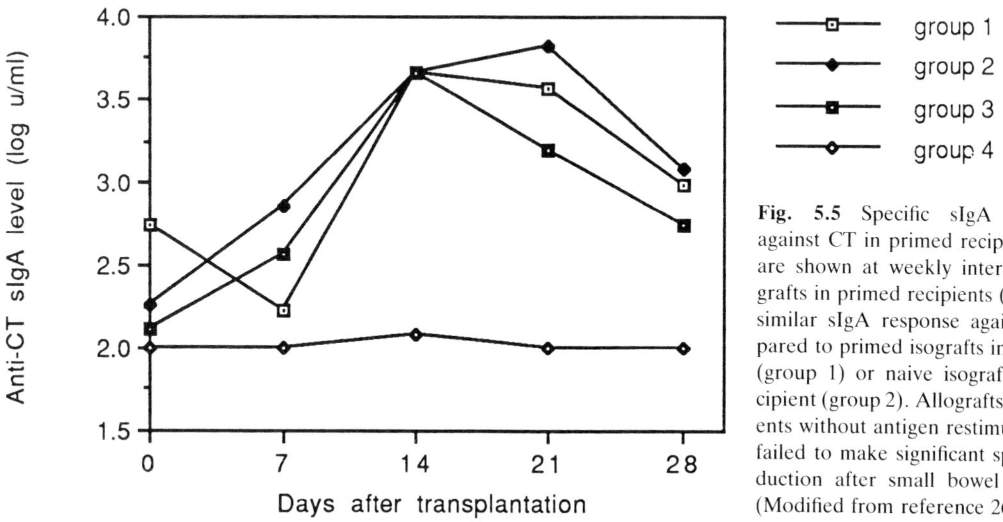

Fig. 5.5 Specific sIgA levels directed against CT in primed recipients (Table 5.4) are shown at weekly intervals. Naive allografts in primed recipients (group 3) made a similar sIgA response against CT as compared to primed isografts in naive recipients (group 1) or naive isografts in primed recipient (group 2). Allografts in primed recipients without antigen restimulation (group 4) failed to make significant specific sIgA production after small bowel transplantation. (Modified from reference 26.)

after transplantation. Significant differences were found at all time points after restimulation when comparing Group 1, 2 or 3 with Group 4 ($p < 0.05$). There was no evidence for rejection in any group.

Inhibitory effect of CsA on specific sIgA production against CT

The reason for the failure of naive transplanted small bowel to make specific sIgA in response to immunization with CT is unclear from the above studies. Since CsA was given only for 7 days and since this short-term CsA both delayed the specific sIgA response in isografts and failed to achieve long-term graft survival in allografts, either CsA or rejection might have caused the unresponsiveness to CT. To separate the effects of CsA from those of rejection on the production of specific sIgA against CT, we designed the following long-term CsA experiment. CsA was administered for four weeks after transplantation to achieve a long surviving allograft model. CT was injected into the graft either during or after CsA treatment and specific sIgA were measured after immunization.

Six groups were studied (Table 5.5). CT (10 μg) was injected intraluminally into the grafts two times, one week apart. Groups 1–3 were immunized at day 0 and 7 when the animals were being given CsA, while groups 4–6 were immunized at days 28 and 35 after completion of the CsA treatment. CsA was administered for 4 weeks at a dose of 15 mg/kg/d for the first week and 10 mg/kg/d for the following 3 weeks.

Table 5.5 Experimental groups with prolonged CsA administration

Group	CsA	CT immunization	n
1 LBNF1->LBNF1	—	day 0 and 7	5
2 LBNF1->LBNF1	day 0–28	day 0 and 7	10
3 LBNF1->Lewis	day 0–28	day 0 and 7	4
4 LBNF1->LBNF1	—	day 28 and 35	9
5 LBNF1->LBNF1	day 0–28	day 28 and 35	9
6 LBNF1->Lewis	day 0–28	day 28 and 35	11

The CsA regimen used in this experiment prevented rejection in all allograft groups until the end of the experiment, thus allowing us to separate the effects of immunosuppression from rejection. No specific sIgA was detected in any group prior to immunization (Fig. 5.6). Non-CsA treated isografts (Group 1) made the expected specific sIgA response to CT after immunization. However, neither isografts (Group 2) nor allografts (Group 3) immunized during long-term CsA treatment made any response against CT. Significant differences were found at all postoperative time points when comparing group 2 or 3 to group 1 ($p < 0.05$). In contrast, specific sIgA was found in all three groups in which immunization was carried out after CsA treatment was completed, as shown in Fig. 5.6. Specific sIgA levels in isografts (Group 4) rose and reached peak level at seven days after the second immunization (day 42) and declined slightly thereafter. Allografts (Group 6) showed a similar pattern of

kinetics, antigen specificity and blocking by anti-Ia antisera. *Immunology* 1986; **58,** 1–7.
3. Bland PW, Warren LG. Antigen presentation by epithelial cells of the rat small bowel intestine II: selective induction of suppressor T cells. *Immunology* 1986; **58,** 9–14.
4. Mayer L, Shlien R. Evidence for function of Ia molecules on gut epithelial cells in man. *J Exp Med* 1987; **166,** 1471–83.
5. Bland P. MHC class II expression by the gut epithelium. *Immunol Today* 1988; **9,** 174–8.
6. Goldblum RM. The role of IgA in local immune protection. *J Clin Immunol* 1990; **10,** 64s–71s.
7. Winer L, Mack J, Weltzin R, Mekalanos JJ, Kraehenbuhl J, Neutra MR. *Infection and Immunity* 1991; **59,** 977–82.
8. Strober W, Sneller MC. IgA deficiency. *Ann Allergy* 1991; **66,** 363–75.
9. Brandtzaeg P. Overview of the mucosal immune system. *Curr Top Microbiol Immunol* 1989; **146,** 13–25.
10. Balk SP, Ebert EE, Blumenthal RL, McDermoot FV. Wucherpfennig K, Landau SB, Blumberg RS. Human intestinal intraepithelial lymphocytes are oligoclonal and recognized CD1. *Science* 1991; **253,** 1411–15.
11. Lefrancois L, Goodman T. In vivo modulation of cytolytic activity and Thy-1 expression in TCR-rq+ intraepithelial lymphocytes. *Science* 1989; **243,** 1716–18.
12. Klein J. Ontogeny of the Thy-, Lyt-2 murine intestinal intraepithelial lymphocyte: characterization of a unique population of thymus-independent cytotoxic effector cells in the intestinal mucosa. *J Exp Med* 1986; **164,** 309–14.
13. Shanahan F, Brogan M, Targan S. Human mucosal cytotoxic effector cells. *Gastroenterology* 1987; **92,** 1951–7.
14. Klein JR, Kagnoff MF. Spontaneous in vitro evolution of lytic specificity of cytotoxic T lymphocyte clones isolated from murine intestinal epithelium. *J Immunol* 1987; **138,** 58–62.
15. Kanof ME, Strober W. Lymphokine-activated killer-cell cytotoxicity in the intestinal immune system. *Gastroenterology* 1989; **97**, 222–4.
16. Tagliabue A, Nencioni L, Villa L, Keren DF, Lowell GH, Boraschi D. Antibody-dependent cell-mediated antibacterial activity of intestinal lymphocytes with secretory IgA. *Nature* 1983; **306,** 184–6.
17. Tagliabue A, Boraschi D, Villa L, Keren DF, Lowell GH, Rappuoli R, Nencioni L. IgA-dependent cell-mediated activity against enteropathogenic bacteria: distribution, specificity, and characterization of the effector cells. *J Immunol* 1984; **133,** 988–92.
18. Mowat AM. The regulation of immune responses to dietary protein antigens. *Immunol Today* 1987; **8**, 93–8.
19. Tomasi TB. Oral tolerance. *Transplantation* 1980; **29,** 353–6.
20. Lamont AG, Mowat AM, Parrott MV. Priming of systemic and local delayed-type hypersensitivity responses by feeding low doses of ovalbumin to mice. *Immunology* 1989; **66,** 595–9.
21. Sayegh MH, Khoury SJ, Hancock WW, Weiner HL, Carpenter CB. Induction of immunity and oral tolerance with polymorphic class II major histocompatibility complex allopeptides in the rat. *Immunology* 1992; **89,** 7762–6.
22. Kirkman RL. Small bowel transplantation. *Transplantation* 1984; **37,** 429–33.
23. Xia W, Kirkman RL. Immune function in transplated small intestine: total secretory IgA production and response against cholera toxin. *Transplantation* 1990; **49,** 277–80.
24. Xia W, Xia SS. Orthotopic and heterotopic small bowel transplantation in rats. *Chin Med J* 1988; **101,** 13–16.
25. Xia W, Kirkman RL. Immune function in transplanted small intestine II: sIgA production in cholera toxin primed rats. *Transplant Proc* 1990; **22,** 2481–2.
26. Xia W, Kirkman RL. Cyclosporine A inhibits specific sIgA production against cholera toxin but not trinitrophynyl-lipopolysaccride (TNP-LPS) in small bowel transplantation. *Transplant Proc* 1992; **24,** 1155–6.
27. Xia W, Kirkman RL. Priming the recipient abrogates the inhibitory effect of CsA on specific sIgA production against cholera toxin in small bowel transplantation. *Transplant Proc* 1992; **24,** 1139–40.
28. Xia W, Kirkman RL. Inhibitory effect of cyclosporine on specific secretory IgA production against cholera toxin in small bowel transplantation. *Transplant Proc* 1991; **23,** 682–3.
29. Madara JL, Kirkman RL. Structure and functional evolation of jejunal allograft rejectionin rats and the ameliorating effects of cyclosporine therapy. *J Clin Invest* 1985; **75,** 502–12.
30. Kirkman RL, Lear PA, Madara JL, Tilney NL. Small bowel transplantation in the rat-immunology and function. *Surgery* 1984; **96,** 280–6.
31. Monchik GJ, Russell PS. Transplantation of small bowel transplantation. *Surgery* 1971; **70,** 693–701.
32. Lear PA, Cunningham AJ, Crane PW, Wood RFM. Lymphocyte migration patterns in small bowel transplants. *Transplant Proc* 1989; **21,** 2881–2.
33. Iwaki Y, Starzl TE, Yagihashi A, Taniwaki S, Abu-Elmagd K, Tzakis A, Fung J, Todo S. Replacement of donor lymphoid tissue in small bowel transplants. *Lancet* 1991; **337,** 818–19.

6

The mucosal barrier

Bradley H Collins and R Randal Bollinger

Introduction

The gastrointestinal tract is a complex organ system whose primary function is the digestion of food and subsequent absorption of nutrients necessary for the maintenance of bodily processes. The intestinal mucosa is continuously exposed to potentially harmful substances in the form of ingested matter and resident flora; therefore, in addition to its digestive function, the gastrointestinal tract must prevent the penetration of these potential pathogens. This ability has been aptly termed the 'mucosal barrier' and has been the subject of intense research. Failure of the barrier has been demonstrated for decades and has been implicated in disease processes ranging from gastrointestinal food allergy to the progression of the multisystem organ failure syndrome.

Transplantation of the small intestine has been attempted for many years; however, only recently has success been realized.[1,2] It is inherent that procedural requirements such as luminal flushing and cold ischaemia have an effect on the mucosal barrier and render the recipient susceptible to complications not commonly observed in the recipients of other types of grafts. This chapter will outline the components of the mucosal barrier, discuss intestinal permeability and bacterial translocation, and describe the effects of experimental small bowel transplantation on mucosal barrier function.

Mucosal barrier

The function of the intestinal mucosal barrier is to prevent the penetration of luminal macromolecules and bacteria through the enterocytes and into the portal blood circulation or lymphatic system (see Table 6.1). Several mechanisms have been proposed to account for the ability of some large molecules and potential pathogens to traverse this continuous membrane layer. These include endocytosis (both receptor-mediated and non-selective), transcellular or direct cellular membrane penetration, and incompetent intercellular junctions (see Fig. 6.1).[3]

The intestinal mucosal barrier is underdeveloped in both human and animal neonates.[4,5] As the neonate matures, the intestinal mucosa becomes less permeable to various macromolecules such as immunoglobulin and ingested proteins; however, prior to the maturity of barrier function, these large molecules are capable of being transported across the mucosa and can be detected in the systemic circulation.[4,5] Endocytosis is the mechanism by which macromolecules gain access to the immature enterocytes.[4] The intracellular vesicles containing these molecules combine with lysosomes and the contents are digested; however, in some instances the macromolecules are not degraded and are then extruded from the cells into the lateral intercellular space via exocytosis. It is at this point that the mucosal barrier has been breached and the foreign antigens can invade the portal circulation or lymphatic system. Immaturity of barrier function is thought to be associated with the pathogenesis of several clinically relevant disorders, including gastrointestinal food allergy and necrotizing enterocolitis.[4] The development of allergies to certain foods is felt by some investigators to be mediated by sensitization to ingested protein antigens that have transgressed an immature barrier. Oral tolerance is a mech-

Table 6.1 Components of the intestinal mucosal barrier

Nonimmunologic Components
Saliva
Gastric Acid
Proteolysis
Peristalsis
Mucus
Flora of the Gastrointestinal Tract
Immunologic Components
Gut-Associated Lymphoid Tissue (GALT)
Peyer's patches
IgA-producing plasma cells of the lamina propria
Hepatic IgA
Biliary IgA derived from serum via hepatobiliary transport

anism that inhibits undesired immune responses to commonly encountered food antigens and, therefore, serves to limit the development of disorders such as food allergies.[6] The clinical syndrome observed in neonates with necrotizing enterocolitis may result from the invasion of the immature intestinal barrier by bacteria and endotoxin. A recent study indicates that the development of insulin-dependent diabetes mellitus in some patients may be mediated by anti-bovine serum album antibodies that cross-react with a protein on the surfaces of pancreatic beta cells.[7] These antibodies, which are formed after ingested cow's milk crosses the intestinal barrier, are capable of damaging beta cells. It is evident that an immature intestinal barrier function plays a role in clinically relevant disorders. Although the mucosal barrier becomes less permeable as the intestines mature, a small amount of macromolecular uptake apparently occurs even after full maturity; however, this appears to be an insignificant, well-controlled, immunologic process.[8]

Saliva

Saliva is the first component of the intestinal barrier system that ingested materials encounter. Although the oral cavity harbours a large population of resident flora, saliva contains multiple factors that serve to limit the adherence and proliferation of bacteria. Lysozyme exerts its antibacterial activity by degrading the bacterial cell wall, whereas lactoferrin depletes the iron supply necessary for microbial survival.[9] Immunoglobulin A (IgA), the immunoglobulin of the

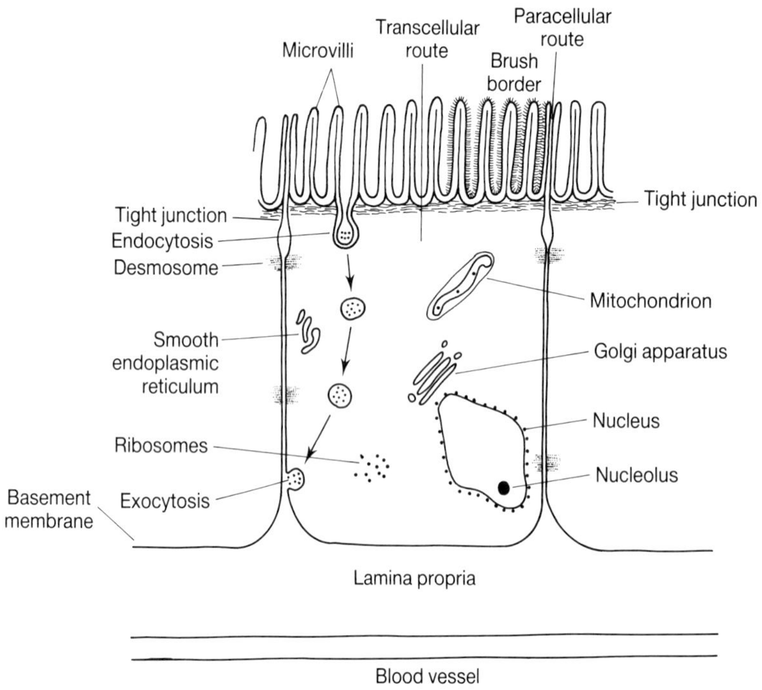

Fig. 6.1 (1) This diagram depicts some mechanisms by which the intestinal mucosal layer may be breached by antigens. Molecules can gain access to the cells via endocytosis at the luminal border. These antigens can then be transported through the enterocytes within a vesicle and deposited via exocytosis near the basement membrane where they can enter the portal circulation. (2) Direct penetration of the cellular membrane has also been reported (transcellular route). (3) Junctions are present within the lateral membranes of enterocytes. *Tight junctions* separate the intestinal lumen from the intercellular spaces and play a major role in maintenance of mucosal integrity by inhibiting paracellular travel. *Gap junctions* permit the intercellular transfer of electrolytes and small molecules.

secretory immune system, is also present in saliva where it contributes to the neutralization of bacteria and viruses.[9]

Gastric acidity

The acidic environment of the stomach contributes to the intestinal barrier. It aids in the digestion of potentially harmful macromolecules, thereby decreasing the amount of material available for penetration of the intestinal mucosa and hence transgression of the barrier.[8] Experimental data supporting the contention that gastric acidity augments the intestinal barrier are provided by Bloch et al. who demonstrated increased intestinal macromolecular transport following neutralization of gastric pH in rats.[10]

The most significant contribution of gastric acid to maintaining the mucosal barrier is the prevention of bacterial colonization of the proximal small intestine.[11] In a healthy individual, the stomach is virtually free of bacteria and the duodenum is considered 'relatively sterile'. However, patients with achlorhydria (the inability of the stomach to secrete hydrochloric acid) often have increased numbers of bacteria in the upper small intestine and, therefore, are possibly at increased risk for acquiring invasive bacterial infections originating in the proximal gastrointestinal tract.[11,12,13]

Like other components of the intestinal barrier, the gastric acid secreting apparatus of the neonatal stomach is immature and develops during the first few weeks of life.[11,14] The result is a 'relative hypochlorhydria' during neonatal development which contributes to the immature barrier function observed in the neonate and leads to increased macromolecular and bacterial uptake across the mucosa.[11]

Proteolysis

The initial steps of protein digestion occur in the stomach where proteins are denatured by gastric acid, thereby subjecting interior peptide bonds to hydrolysis by pepsin.[15] Proteolysis by pepsin is a limited process because as the gastric contents exit the stomach, the activity of this peptidase is terminated by the higher pH encountered in the duodenum.[16] Most proteolysis occurs in the small intestine where pancreatic enzymes digest proteins to free amino acids and short peptides.[16] Intestinal brush-border enzymes are also involved in the digestion of proteins.[16] The subsequent absorption of amino acids and short peptides by enterocytes occurs by a variety of mechanisms that range from simple diffusion to carrier-mediated systems.[15,16]

Proteins that escape complete digestion may be transported across the intestinal barrier in the form of antigenic macromolecules and gain access to the lymphatic system or systemic circulation. The enhanced ability of preterm neonates to absorb ingested milk antigens has been attributed to the presence of an immature intestinal barrier.[17] The decreased level of intestinal proteolysis observed in neonates by some investigators probably contributes to this effect.[4] Utilizing an experimental model, Udall et al. demonstrated that the inhibition of pancreatic enzymes resulted in increased uptake of macromolecules across the intestinal barrier.[18] This evidence supports the theory that proteolysis contributes to barrier function by limiting the quantity of macromolecular substances available for transport across the barrier.

Peristalsis

Small intestinal peristalsis certainly plays a role in maintaining the mucosal barrier and is even considered by some to be the most significant factor in containing bacterial colonization of the small intestine.[11] The ability of potential pathogens such as bacteria and antigenic macromolecules to associate with enterocytes is hindered by peristalsis which propels luminal contents along the gastrointestinal tract. Segments of intestine that exhibit hypomotility are subject to a phenomenon known as the 'blind loop syndrome' or the 'contaminated small bowel syndrome'.[11,19] The luminal contents of hypomotile lengths of intestine are prone to stasis which produces an environment that is conducive to bacterial overgrowth.[20] Microscopic evaluation of hypomotile segments of small bowel harbouring bacterial overgrowth reveals a characteristic mucosal lesion that possibly provides a portal of entry for antigenic molecules.[8,20] Normal peristalsis fortifies the intestinal barrier by controlling bacterial proliferation and limiting the opportunity for macromolecules to associate with enterocytes and cross the barrier. It is likely that the hypomotility observed in the neonatal small intestine contributes to the immature barrier.[4]

Mucus

The layer of mucus that covers the epithelial surface of the gastrointestinal tract is a physical component of the intestinal barrier that bacteria and macromolecular antigens encounter prior to gaining access to the mucous membrane. It is produced by epithelial goblet cells and then secreted into the lumen. The ability of peristalsis to propel bacteria and other potential pathogens is greatly enhanced by the presence of mucus that serves to lubricate luminal surfaces and contents.[3] Mucin is the viscous form of mucus that lines the epithelial surface and is composed of glycoproteins and glycolipids.[4,8] It has been shown to interfere with the attachment of bacteria to the epithelial cells, thereby limiting their ability to transgress the intestinal barrier.[4] The interaction of bacteria with the epithelial surface is via 'receptors' on the mucosal cells that are composed of carbohydrate complexes.[4] The glycoprotein component of mucin contains carbohydrate structures that are analogous to those on the mucosal cells. As bacteria migrate through the intestine, the mucinous glycoproteins adhere to the surfaces of the microbes and inhibit their ability to interact with the mucosal 'receptors'.[14] Many substances that are potential pathogens, such as bacterial toxins or food antigens, have been shown to stimulate the release of mucin under certain experimental conditions.[21,22] It thus appears that, in addition to the standard layer of mucin that lines the intestinal tract, additional amounts may be recruited to augment the barrier when necessary.

As with other components of the intestinal barrier, neonates probably exhibit some deficiencies in the mucous layer that contribute to barrier immaturity. After comparing the intestinal mucus of neonatal rats to that of adults, Shub et al. discovered physical and compositional differences in the glycoproteins.[23] Some have hypothesized that these differences result in decreased adherence of bacteria to the mucin layer, thereby favouring attachment of the microorganisms to intestinal mucosal cells of neonates.[4]

Flora

The resident flora of the intestines exert a significant influence in preventing colonization of the gastrointestinal tract by pathogens. The intestines are sterile at birth; however, bacterial colonization begins by the second day and approximates the composition of adult flora within several weeks (see Table 6.2).[11] Studies of neonates with complete intestinal obstruction secondary to atresia reveal that bacteria are present in the small bowel proximal to the obstruction; however, the distal small intestine is sterile.[24] This finding indicates that the small intestine is populated by ingested microbes and not by organisms inhabiting the colon. The flora of the normal host in the fasting state is a stable population of assorted bacteria and fungi.[11,25] The acidic environment of the stomach makes it an unsuitable place for bacterial proliferation, and in fact, it is 'virtually sterile'.[11] The duodenum and proximal jejunum are considered relatively sterile and harbour 10^3 to 10^4 microorganisms per millilitre of aspirate.[11] Typical organisms inhabiting the proximal small intestine include aerobic bacteria, especially gram-positive species, and yeasts.[11] Cultures of jejunal aspirates obtained from healthy individuals do not grow bacteria in approximately 35 per cent of cases.[25] The microbial burden gradually increases along the small intestine such that the terminal ileum contains 10^5 to 10^8 microorganisms per millilitre of aspirate.[11] Coliforms, such as *Escherichia coli* and *Pseudomonas* species, and anaerobes are present in the distal small intestine.[12,20] The bacterial population of the colon includes 10^8 aerobic microorganisms and 10^9 to 10^{11} anaerobic microorganisms per gram of stool.[11] The aerobes include coliforms and the anaerobes include such species as *Bacteriodes* and *Clostridia*.[11]

The interplay of several mechanisms is probably responsible for the ability of the resident flora to inhibit the proliferation of pathogenic microbes. Theories that have been proposed include the production of an environment not con-

Table 6.2 Bacterial content of the gastrointestinal tract

Location	Microorganisms per Milliliter of Aspirate
Stomach	virtually sterile
Duodenum	10^3–10^4
Proximal Jejunum	10^3–10^4
Terminal Ileum	10^5–10^8
Colon	10^8 aerobic organisms, 10^9–10^{11} anaerobic organisms

ducive to the proliferation of pathogens, the synthesis of antibacterial agents by normal resident species, and the depletion of nutrients necessary for pathogen growth.[3] Circumstances that bring about a change in the normal intestinal ecology may result in the overgrowth of certain resident or pathogenic microorganisms and place the host at risk for infections. Another complication is the translocation of bacteria and their toxins across the intestinal barrier and subsequent invasion of the lymphatic system or systemic circulation. The translocation phenomenon will be addressed in a later section.

Gut-Associated Lymphoid Tissues (GALT)

The term gut-associated lymphoid tissues (GALT) refers to the collection of immune structures and cells that comprise the immunologic system of the gastrointestinal tract. The submucosa of the small intestine contains aggregates of lymphoid cells termed 'Peyer's patches'. Some of these are present in the jejunum; however, the majority are located in the ileum. The 'dome' of an individual Peyer's patch is immediately below the intestinal epithelial layer and contains various cells including T and B lymphocytes and macrophages.[4] The surface of the dome is lined by membranous epithelial cells called M cells.[4] Experimental evidence indicates that M cells may play a role in antigen uptake and presentation.[26] In addition to penetrating the mucosal barrier via the enterocytes and intercellular junctions, it is possible that antigenic macromolecules may gain access to the lymphatic system through interactions with the M cells.[8,26]

'Intraepithelial lymphocytes', as their name implies, are located within the epithelial layer of the intestine. These cells are adjacent to enterocytes; however, tight junctions do not exist between the two types of cells.[4] Most intraepithelial lymphocytes are T cells, 90 per cent of which are of the CD8+ (suppressor/cytotoxic) variety.[27] Although their function is unknown, intraepithelial lymphocytes may contribute to mucosal barrier function by suppressing the local immune responses elicited by antigens that evade other intestinal barrier defence mechanisms.[28]

As with other regions of the secretory immune system, IgA is the primary immunoglobulin of the intestinal mucosa. In humans the majority is produced by plasma cells that reside in the lamina propria; however, hepatic plasma cells synthesize a small amount that reaches the intestinal lumen via the bile.[29] Additional biliary IgA is obtained from the systemic circulation via hepatobiliary transport.[29] Intestinal IgA is a dimer that is linked covalently by a peptide produced by plasma cells called the J chain.[4] Transport of IgA across the epithelial cells into the lumen is facilitated by the binding of the peptide secretory component to the IgA dimers, thus producing secretory IgA (sIgA).[6] Due to its dimeric structure and the presence of the bound peptides, sIgA is relatively resistant to the proteolytic enzymes in the small intestine.[4] Secretory IgA contributes to the intestinal barrier by binding bacteria and other potential pathogens and, thereby, prevents their interaction with and penetration of epithelial cells.[46] It is also thought that some of the ingested proteins that are potentially antigenic macromolecules capable of penetrating the mucosal barrier are bound by sIgA and then enzymatically digested.[6]

The immaturity noted in the neonatal intestinal barrier is certainly multifactorial. Perkkiö et al. have shown that for almost the first two weeks of human life, cells containing immunoglobulin cannot be demonstrated in the intestine.[30] Although breast-fed babies passively receive IgA from ingested colostrum, the absence of native intestinal IgA may contribute to the increased uptake of macromolecules across the immature barrier. The effect of the absence of IgA on the host has been studied in individuals with selective IgA deficiency. These individuals are not prone to gastrointestinal infections; however, circulating antigen-antibody complexes and antibodies to food proteins have been demonstrated in some of them.[6,31]

Intestinal permeability

Intestinal permeability is defined as 'the facility with which the . . . mucosal surface can be penetrated by the unmediated diffusion of specific constituents in a given period'.[32] This 'unmediated diffusion' across the epithelial layer can occur through channels in the enterocytes or via intercellular pathways.[32] Investigators have demonstrated that intestinal epithelial cells are capable of excluding small molecules with radii of 3 angstroms (Å); however, molecules one order of magnitude larger, such as albumin (radius = 36 Å), have also been shown to be capable of crossing this apparently intact layer of cells.[33] The presence of two classes of transmembrane pores, small (radius = to 7 Å) and large (radius at least 65 Å), accounts for these findings.[33] The movement of molecules between enterocytes is regulated by the junctions that exist in the lateral surfaces of the cell membranes (see Fig 6.1).[32] Tight junctions are located just below the layer of microvilli and represent the areas of fusion between the lateral membranes of adjacent mucosal cells.[32,34] These junctions are barricades that separate the intestinal lumen from the intercellular spaces; therefore, their integrity is a major determinant of competent barrier function.[32] Additional types of junctions situated in the lateral cell membrane include adhering junctions that play a role in linking epithelial cells together and gap junctions that allow the intercellular transfer of electrolytes and small molecules.[32]

For the purposes of this discussion, increased intestinal permeability is defined as the excessive or abnormal passage of molecules across the epithelial layer secondary to barrier failure. There are many clinical conditions that are associated with increased intestinal permeability to selected agents. The majority of disorders result in demonstrable mucosal lesions; therefore, it is likely that the increased permeability is due to the movement of molecules through and between damaged enterocytes. Although it is obvious that prolonged interruption in small intestinal blood flow ultimately results in mucosal death and the massive transfer of luminal molecules and bacteria across the barrier, a significant reduction in blood flow produces mucosal layer lesions capable of rendering the barrier incompetent. Chiu et al. were able to show the consistent development of 'space' beneath jejunal and ileal epithelial cells in dogs subjected to an acute 60 to 70 per cent reduction in superior mesenteric artery flow after only 30 minutes.[35] This space, also known as Gruenhagen's space, develops when epithelial cells separate from the basement membrane and is easily detected with light microscopy.[35] It should be emphasized that Gruenhagen's space occurs so early in the course of ischaemic epithelial injury that the epithelial cells are still biochemically functional.[35] Prolonged reduction in blood flow results in progression of the mucosal lesions such that villus capillaries are eventually exposed to luminal contents and bacteria.[35] Granger et al. utilized the plasma-to-lumen clearance of various solutes to assess intestinal epithelial layer integrity.[33] Utilization of this method requires one to envision the mucosal barrier in reverse in that the test agents are placed into the bloodstream at known concentrations, and their clearance into the intestinal lumen is measured. The plasma-to-lumen clearance has been shown to be a function of mucosal barrier integrity. For example, in ischaemia/reperfusion studies of canine intestine, Granger et al. demonstrated an increase in albumin clearance that was proportional to the length and degree of ischaemia and correlated with the histological grade of mucosal damage.[33] Experimental evidence indicates that in the case of transient ischaemia, the reperfusion injury that ultimately results in the barrier damage is possibly mediated by xanthine oxidase.[33] Xanthine metabolism produces hydrogen peroxide and superoxide which generate hydroxyl radicals.[33] These radicals cause lipid peroxidation of cell membranes, and the subsequent inflammation attracts neutrophils which are also capable of effecting cellular injury via the actions of noxious agents including oxidants and proteases.[33] As is evident from the preceding discussion, intestinal ischaemia induces mucosal disruption by a variety of mechanisms and hence is one of the etiologies of barrier failure.

Although increased intestinal permeability can be demonstrated in patients with intestinal ischaemia, results of permeability testing in individuals in whom the diagnosis is being ruled out have no current clinical value. The decision to operate depends on the presence of an acute abdomen or evidence of superior mesenteric artery occlusion on angiography. Despite this specific drawback, permeability testing has proven clinically useful for a number of other conditions affecting the small intestine. Athough several agents are currently employed for these studies, none is considered ideal. 'The ideal passive permeability marker should be nontoxic, hydrophilic, lipophobic, absorbed entirely by passive diffusion, not modified by enzymes, not in the diet, not produced endogenously, not metabolized, excreted rapidly and completely, limited to the extracellular compartment, and easily measurable in body fluids.'[36] Chromium-labelled ethylenediaminetetra-acetate (^{51}Cr-EDTA) is frequently used because only a small amount is absorbed by the normal intestine. This radioactive substance has a molecular radius of 6.8 Å and readily crosses endothelial cells of the villus capillaries thus gaining access to the systemic circulation once the layer of epithelial cells has been breached.[33] Following oral administration in the presence of increased permeability, ^{51}Cr-EDTA crosses the intestinal barrier and reaches the systemic circulation. Clearance is dependent on glomerular filtration; therefore, complete urine collection is necessary for adequate analysis of results. Polyethylene glycol (PEG) is an agent available in a variety of sizes that is also used for permeability testing and can also be administered orally. Although permeability tests with PEG are somewhat difficult to analyse due to the requirement for high-performance liquid chromatography to measure it in the urine, the utilization of two distinct sizes of PEG allows clinicians to correct for factors that do not necessarily relate to small intestinal permeability.[32] These include transit time, dilution within the gastrointestinal tract, and delayed gastric emptying (perhaps secondary to gastroparesis or gastric outlet obstruction).[32] The utilization of two agents at known concentrations enables one to determine the ratio present in the urine.[32] In theory, the extraneous variables outlined above affect both agents equally; therefore, the excretion ratio remains unchanged and any abnormality in the ratio should reflect abnormal permeability. Permeability tests have also been performed with sugar combinations. Sugars such as mannitol, rhamnose, lactulose, and cellobiose have been employed for such studies.[37]

Abnormalities in small intestinal permeability have been noted in a variety of disease processes. Attempts have been made to utilize these tests in the diagnosis and intermittent monitoring of affected patients. Small intestinal permeability has probably been utilized most in the study of individuals with celiac disease. This condition affects the jejunum and is thought to be an immunologically mediated process that has been shown to improve both clinically and histologically when gluten is excluded from the diet. Patients affected with this disease present from infancy to adulthood with a variety of symptoms including diarrhoea and weight loss. The histological findings of this disease are significant for what is termed 'flat jejunal mucosa'.[38] This appearance is due to the absence of villi and a brush border that is underdeveloped or even absent.[38] The epithelial layer is composed of cuboidal cells instead of the normal columnar variety.[38] These mucosal abnormalities resolve when a gluten-free diet is consumed.[38] The diagnosis of celiac disease is a three stage process: 1) jejunal biopsy demonstrating the presence of flat mucosa on histological examination; 2) resolution of the mucosal changes when a gluten-free diet is consumed; 3) and recurrence of the characteristic mucosal lesion when gluten is returned to the diet.[39] Because the diagnosis and monitoring of patients with celiac disease requires at least three jejunal biopsies, investigators have proposed the utilization of permeability testing in an attempt to decrease the number of biopsies performed especially in pediatric patients, a population in whom this procedure is poorly tolerated. Several types of agents have been utilized to assess the intestinal permeability of individuals with celiac disease. The excretion ratio of two orally administered sugars has been frequently employed for these studies.[40–42] Although the results are reported as ratios, interesting results are noted if one considers the urinary excretion of the individual sugars. In patients with untreated celiac disease, investigators have noted that the excretion of small sugars (e.g. mannitol and rhamnose) is significantly reduced as compared to controls, whereas the excretion of disaccharides (e.g. lactulose and cellobiose) is significantly increased.[40–42] It is thought that because the small sugars probably cross the intestinal barrier via pores within the enterocytes, the reduced absorptive area in patients with celiac disease impairs the uptake of these molecules.[40] Disaccharides, on the other hand, probably penetrate the epithelial layer via the tight junctions which are likely to be less competent in celiac disease patients with an abnormal mucosal surface.[40] Other investigators have employed orally administered ^{51}Cr-EDTA to study patients with celiac disease and have reported a significant increase in urinary excretion.[43] Although the reports are somewhat contradictory, abnormalities in intestinal permeability to polyethylene glycols of various sizes probably exist in patients with celiac disease.[44]

In addition to celiac disease, a number of other illnesses are associated with increased small intestinal permeability. Inflammatory bowel disease, specifically Crohn's disease of the small intestine, adversely affects mucosal integrity and leads to increased permeability.[45,46] In fact, Howden et al. were able to demonstrate a correlation between the urinary excretion of orally administered ^{51}Cr-EDTA and the clinical severity of inflammation as determined by common laboratory studies.[46] Additional clinical conditions that have been shown to be associated with increased small intestinal permeability as demonstrated by the test agents discussed above include chronic renal failure, non-steroidal anti-inflammatory drug use, burn-related infections, and cow's milk intolerance.[47–50]

Bacterial translocation

The term bacterial translocation refers to the penetration of viable bacteria and bacterial products (e.g. endotoxin) through the epithelial layer of the gastrointestinal tract to the mesenteric lymph nodes and other organ systems. Although bacterial translocation has only recently become the subject of considerable research, this phenomenon has been recognized for at least a century with reports in the German literature documenting the passage of viable bacteria through apparently intact intestinal mucosa.[51] In the 1920s, Arnold and Brody demonstrated that bacteria injected into the duodenums of normal dogs could be detected in the effluent of the thoracic duct if the bacteria were administered in an alkaline solution in the presence of a foreign antigen.[52] Fine et al. are credited with determining the clinical relevance of what was then termed 'transmural migration'.[53] The use of the word translocation to describe this process is attributed to Keller and Engley who used this word in their assessment of the 'fate of bacteriophage particles introduced into mice' via the gastrointestinal tract.[54]

In order for bacteria and endotoxins to gain access to the lymphatic system and/or the systemic circulation, violation of the gastrointestinal tract's mucosal barrier must occur. It has become increasingly apparent that in clinically relevant bacterial translocation, indigenous organisms that comprise the resident flora (also known as the autochthonous flora) penetrate the mucosal barrier and are subsequently responsible for the infectious complications and hemodynamic derangements associated with this phenomenon. This section will not address the passage of 'foreign' pathogenic bacteria across the mucosal barrier but will focus on the passage of indigenous organisms. The components of the mucosal barrier outlined previously, both immunologic and non-immunologic, are responsible for maintaining normal intraluminal ecology; however, various clinical syndromes and physiologic alterations can lead to barrier failure and subsequent bacterial translocation. Although different organisms probably employ distinct mechanisms to transgress the mucosal layer, bacteria and endotoxin very likely cross the epithelial layer either by direct cellular penetration or via intercellular pathways. The exact mechanism by which bacteria reach the lymphatic system and systemic circulation is not known; however, theories have been proposed. For example, Wells et al. have hypothesized that following penetration of the epithelial layer, it is likely that bacteria are ingested by mobile phagocytic cells (probably macrophages) located in the Peyer's patches and lamina propria.[55] Peyer's patches are lymphocyte collections that are located in the submucosa. Small intestinal lymphatic effluent drains into a series of mesenteric lymph nodes, then into larger intestinal lymphatics, then into the cisterna chyli, and finally into the thoracic duct. The thoracic duct drains into the origin of the left internal jugular or innominate vein, thus completing the course from the intestinal lumen to the systemic circulation. Following ingestion of bacteria, the phagocytes are capable of transporting the bacteria to the lymphatic system or systemic circulation; however, due to failure of intracellular killing mechanisms and the subsequent death of the phagocytes, viable bacteria are deposited in extraintestinal locations.[55] It is also possible that bacteria gain access to the systemic circulation by invasion of the intestinal blood vessels which drain into the portal venous system. The liver is capable of clearing bacteria due to the phagocytic activity of Kupffer cells; however, if it is overwhelmed, then systemic invasion can occur.

There is a large body of experimental evidence that implicates bacterial translocation in the pathogenesis of a number of clinical processes. For example, most deaths that occur in trauma patients who survive more than two days are the result of sepsis.[56] In fact, the organisms responsible for the infectious complications in a significant number of these patients are normal inhabitants of the gastrointestinal tract.[56] Utilizing as a working hypothesis the fact that bacteria can migrate across the intestinal barrier, investigators have generated a number of experimental conditions that mimic the clinical situations thought to be conducive to bacterial translocation. Baker et al. have demonstrated the phenomenon of bacterial translocation in rats subjected to haemorrhagic shock.[56] They were even able to show a correlation between the quantity of bacteria cultured from the mesenteric lymph nodes and the duration of ischaemia. Deitch et al. demonstrated that inhibition of the xanthine oxidase system significantly reduced the incidence of bacterial translocation to the mesenteric lymph nodes in rats subjected to haemorrhagic shock followed by the reinfusion of the removed blood.[57] They concluded that the increase in bacterial translocation associated with haemorrhagic shock was likely due to barrier injury mediated by the oxygen-free radicals released by the xanthine oxidase system upon reperfusion. It is logical that an intact immune system is necessary to maintain the intestinal mucosal barrier. One of the major complications of chemotherapeutic agents is the state of immunosuppression produced in the recipient and the subsequent susceptibility to infectious complications. In an attempt to study this particular problem, Berg administered various chemotherapeutic agents to specific pathogen-free mice.[58] One week after the drugs had been given, the mesenteric lymph nodes, liver, and spleen of each animal were cultured for bacteria. The incidence of positive cultures was significantly increased in the mice receiving chemotherapeutic agents. The bacteria cultured from these organs were consistent with the gastrointestinal flora of these mice, thereby demonstrating the importance of an intact immune system in preventing bacterial translocation. The importance of a stable indigenous bacterial population in maintaining gastrointestinal mucosal barrier has been stressed in a previous section. The administration of enteral antibiotics can alter the balance of intestinal organisms and allow overgrowth of certain populations. Berg showed that the overgrowth of organisms actually enhanced their propensity to translocate.[59] In his specific pathogen-free mouse model, the administration of penicillin, clindamycin, or metronidazole resulted in bacterial overgrowth of gram-negative enteric bacilli and promoted the translocation of these species to the mesenteric lymph nodes. Total parenteral nutrition (TPN) is utilized to sustain patients unable to maintain adequate enteral nutritional balance because of small intestinal absence or malfunction (e.g. short bowel syndrome, prolonged ileus). Just a few years ago, patients receiving long-term TPN therapy routinely developed reductions in small intestinal mucosal mass that were originally attributed to 'disuse atrophy'. It is plausible that this atrophy of the small intestinal mucosa resulted in disruption of the barrier which possibly enhanced bacterial translocation. Alverdy et al. demonstrated a significant increase in bacterial translocation, as indicated by positive mesenteric lymph node cultures, in rats receiving intravenous hyperalimentation.[60] They theorized that the previously described TPN-induced reduction in secretory IgA levels allowed bacteria increased access to the enterocytes and thus enhanced translocation. It was recently determined that the atrophy associated with TPN is actually due to the absence of glutamine, a primary energy source of the enterocytes, in the TPN solution. In addition to preventing small intestinal mucosal atrophy, the addition of glutamine to intravenous hyperalimentation administered to rats significantly decreased the incidence of bacterial translocation associated with TPN solutions without glutamine.[61]

There are additional experimental models of bacterial translocation that have clinical relevance. Wells et al. produced intra-abdominal abscesses in rats by implanting fibrin clots contaminated with specific bacteria into their peritoneal cavities.[62] Seven days after implantation the abscesses were excised using aseptic technique and cultured. Bacteria originally placed in the clots and additional organisms consistent with the flora of the intestinal tract were subsequently cultured. Control cultures of fibrin clots in rats receiving sterile clots yielded no organisms up to 7 days after implantation. In a somewhat similar study, Mora et al. implanted assorted sterile prosthetic materials into the peritoneal cavities of mice and cultured these items at various time intervals.[63] In addition to the appearance of bacteria consistent with intestinal flora in the implanted biomaterials, they noted the presence of fluorescent beads (1 μm in diameter) which had been placed in the drinking water of the mice. Mora et al. also correlated the appearance of bacteria in the prosthetic materials with their synchronous appearance in the mesenteric lymph nodes. The fluorescent beads were observed in prosthetic materials, as previously stated, and also in the enterocytes and within macrophages of the lamina propria. Taking into account all of the findings, the investigators theorized that the presence of a peri-intestinal focus of inflammation promotes phagocytosis of intestinal bacteria by macrophages which are then attracted to the site of inflammation by chemotaxis. If the macrophages fail to kill the ingested bacteria, then successful translocation of viable organisms to distant sites has occurred. Although many other experimental models of bacterial translocation bearing clinical relevance exist, only one other will be addressed in this section. Endotoxin is a class of lipopolysaccharide molecules with systemic effects synthesized by gram-negative bacteria and, therefore, present in large quantities in the distal gastrointestinal tract. Experimental studies have shown that in addition to crossing the intestinal mucosal barrier, endotoxin is capable of increasing intestinal permeability and even promoting bacterial translocation.[64] Deitch et al. demonstrated the enhancement of bacterial translocation in mice administered endotoxin from *Escherichia coli.*[64] Mesenteric lymph node cultures of those animals receiving intramuscular or intraperitoneal endotoxin revealed the presence of common intestinal bacterial species that comprise the indigenous flora of mice. The role of bacterial and endotoxin translocation in the initiation and perpetuation of disease continues to be defined in the laboratory.

Although there are extensive experimental data documenting the occurrence of bacterial translocation in situations similar to those encountered clinically, the application of this knowledge to the practice of medicine is in the early stages. Controversy exists as to the clinical relevance of bacterial translocation. Based upon extensive experimental data, Deitch has selected three conditions known to promote bacterial translocation in experimental models that probably play a role in human disease: loss of physical integrity of the mucosal barrier, impaired immune function, and bacterial overgrowth.[65]

Patients who experience hypotension, either episodic or prolonged, sustain some element of hypoperfusion of the small intestine. If the reduction in circulation is significant enough, then the patient is at risk for developing mucosal lesions (see Intestinal Permeability), thus rendering the mucosal barrier incompetent. The presence of intestinal hypoperfusion and the subsequent development of mucosal disruption produce a clinical setting conducive to bacterial translocation and its many ramifications. It is interesting to note that not all investigators consider the movement of bacteria across a damaged epithelial layer translocation.[51] Some feel that this represents movement due to increased permeability and not classic translocation which they define as the bacteria transgressing a seemingly intact mucosa. Nevertheless, it is likely that translocation of intestinal bacteria plays a role in the systemic infections noted in victims of severe trauma and other hypotension-inducing conditions (e.g., gram-negative rod septicemia and *Pseudomonas* or *Klebsiella* pneumonia). In addition to causing infectious complications, gram-negative organisms produce endotoxin which contributes to the production of the clinical signs and symptoms associated with the septic state and can exert its effects, such as hypotension, in the absence of a septic focus.[66] It is also likely that endotoxin potentiates, or at least facilitates, bacterial translocation. O'Dwyer et al. were able to demonstrate increased intestinal permeability in normal human volunteers administered a single intravenous dose of *Escherichia coli* endotoxin.[66] This finding establishes the possibility of a vicious cycle in already compromised patients: the presence of extraintestinal endotoxin enhances bacterial translocation which, in turn, increases circulating endotoxin levels which further enhances bacterial translocation. Endotoxin is also thought to contribute to the multiple organ failure syndrome observed in some critically ill patients.[65] For example, there are patients who do not have microbiological evidence of infection who develop multisystem organ failure and subsequently die of what appears to be sepsis.[65] It has been postulated that failure of the intestinal mucosal barrier permits endotoxin to enter the portal venous and systemic circulations from which it initiates and perpetuates the septic-like syndrome, including failure of organ systems.[65] Monoclonal antibody (MoAb) therapy has recently been utilized to offset the effects of endotoxin in patients with sepsis due to gram-negative organisms.[67,68] Although the use of these agents is controversial at present, the early indication is that administration of anti-endotoxin MoAb may be beneficial for selected subgroups of patients. For example, treatment with E5 (a murine monoclonal IgM antibody) resulted in significant resolution of organ failure and reduction in mortality in those patients with gram-negative sepsis not associated with shock.[67] The use of HA-1A (a human monoclonal IgM antibody) was associated with decreased mortality in patients with gram-negative bacteraemia whether or not shock was present; however, no benefit was noted in patients with gram-negative infections that were not associated with bacteraemia.[68]

The second factor that Deitch has associated with bacterial translocation is a defect in the immune system.[65] It is well known that patients treated with chemotherapeutic or immunosuppressive agents are at increased risk for developing systemic infections. Some of these infections are caused by organisms also found in the gastrointestinal tract and are likely to be due to bacterial translocation enhanced by incomplete immune function. Owens and Berg demonstrated the presence of viable, enteric bacterial species in the mesenteric lymph nodes and other organs of congenitally athymic mice that significantly exceeded the levels found in control animals.[69] Congenitally athymic mice that received thymic allografts exhibited a translocation rate that was significantly reduced and approximated that of controls. These investigators theorized that T cell-mediated immunity is important in preventing bacterial translocation to the mesenteric lymph nodes and further spread to other tissues. It is likely that suppression of the immune system adversely affects barrier function at multiple levels. Malnutrition may enhance bacterial translocation by the suppressive effect it exerts on the immune system.

Deitch's third factor promoting bacterial translocation is an alteration in the intestinal flora resulting in overgrowth of specific species.[65] Many interventions commonly employed in the treatment of severely ill patients adversely affect the microbial balance of the gastrointestinal tract thereby favouring the overgrowth of some species. The overabundance of a species enhances its likelihood of translocation. The administration of broad-spectrum antibiotics often produces an environment that favours the overgrowth of certain species while inhibiting the growth of others. The use of antacids and type 2 histamine receptor antagonists impairs the gastric acid component of the mucosal barrier which can alter the bacterial population and possibly lead to bacterial overgrowth.[65] In a clinical study that demonstrated bacterial translocation outside the laboratory setting, Deitch cultured mesenteric lymph nodes obtained at abdominal exploration of patients with intestinal obstruction and found a 59 per cent incidence of positive cultures (enteric species) as opposed to 4 per cent positive in patients undergoing laparotomy for other indications.[70] It is not feasible to obtain tissue for culturing in most human disease processes in which bacterial translocation is implicated; however, Deitch converted a common clinical situation into an ingenious model and was able to confirm the presence of translocating bacteria.

Some investigators have proposed 'selective gut decontamination' as a method of reducing the load of gram-negative bacteria in the intestinal tracts of severely ill patients at risk for sepsis.[65] Enterally administered, non-absorbable antibiotics, similar to those that are utilized for preoperative bowel preparations, are employed. This prophylactic removal of bacteria before they translocate is controversial since no survival benefit has been consistently demonstrated.[65]

Small bowel transplantation

Only recently has clinical transplantation of the small intestine been considered more than experimental.[1,2] The initial failures were due to such complications as rejection, infection and technical difficulties.[1] Improvements in immunosuppressive agents, antibiotics, and surgical techniques have enabled surgeons to utilize this operation in the successful treatment of short bowel syndrome.[2] Transplantation of the small intestine raises some interesting issues that relate to mucosal barrier function. The various manipulations necessary for harvesting, preserving, and implanting the small intestine are likely to impair some of the components of the barrier thereby rendering the host susceptible to complications unique to small bowel transplantation.

Graft barrier function

The literature relating barrier function to small bowel transplantation is somewhat limited due to the recently renewed interest in both fields. It is probable that some of the interventions that are necessary for graft implantation are injurious to the mucosa. For example, ischaemia and reperfusion have been shown to damage the intestinal mucosa in experimental models. Ischaemia is an inevitable component of small bowel transplantation and can produce enterocyte damage ranging from the development of Gruenhagen's space, a relatively minor change (see Intestinal Permeability), to severe damage consisting of denuded villi with ulcer formation.[35] Reperfusion is also thought by some investigators to induce barrier damage through the actions of oxygen-free radicals that are generated by the xanthine oxidase system.[57] Physical integrity of the enterocyte layer is an important constituent of the mucosal barrier. Any significant damage to the mucosal cells may weaken the barrier, thereby increasing the patient's risk of bacterial translocation and the subsequent development of infection. The potential complications associated with a damaged mucosa require surgeons to select an adequate storage solution and to limit cold ischaemic time. The mucosal barrier may also be damaged by the host's immune response elicited by the allograft. The effects of rejection on the epithelial layer of the allograft can be readily demonstrated by histology (see Fig. 6.2).

In addition to physical integrity, other components of the barrier system are probably affected by small bowel transplantation. As previously outlined, peristalsis is thought to play a major role in mucosal barrier function by limiting bacterial proliferation. The effect of small bowel transplantation on graft peristalsis is multifactorial. Ileus secondary to manipulation of the graft probably affects bowel motility early in the postoperative course. Although the central nervous system regulates bowel motility through the

(A)

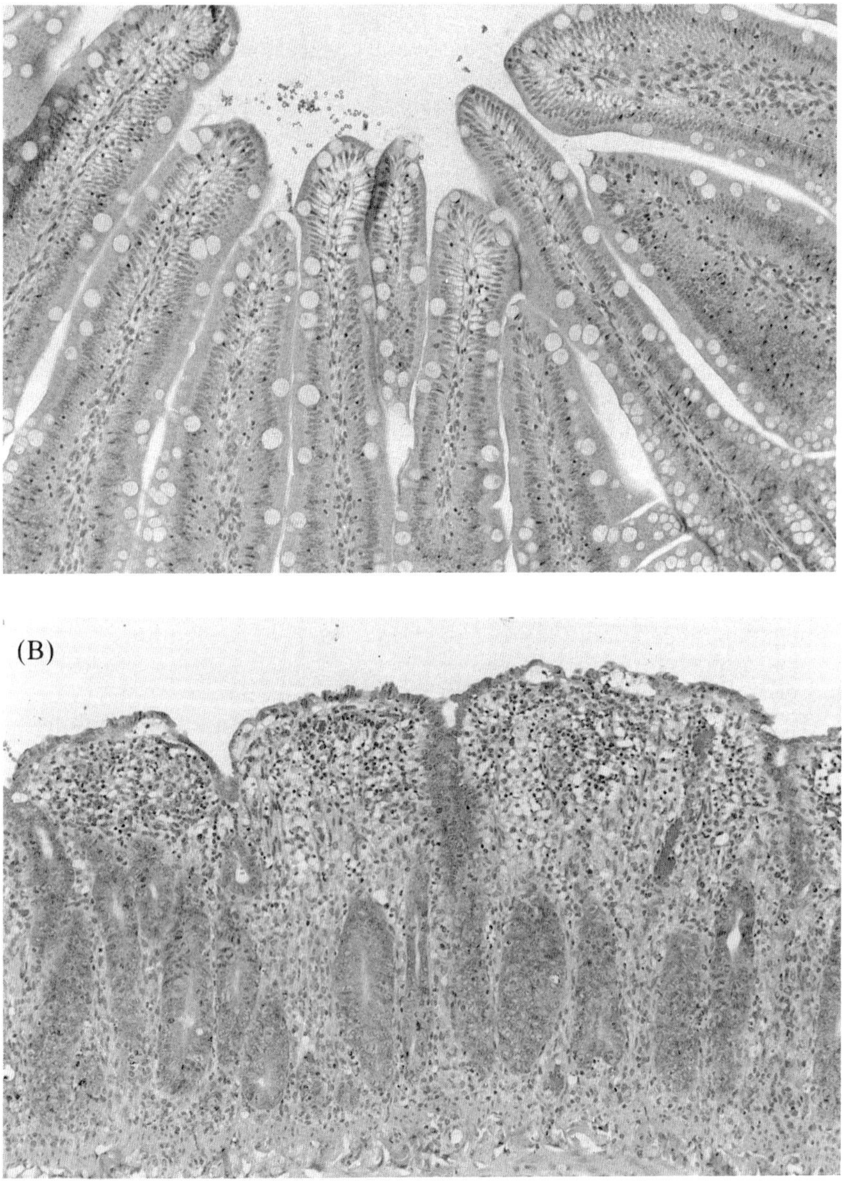

(B)

Fig. 6.2 Small intestinal allografts were performed in rats, and samples of donor ileum were assessed by light microscopy after staining with hematoxylin and eosin (magnification ×140). (A) Adequate postoperative immunosuppression resulted in preservation of villous architecture in this specimen. (B) This specimen reveals signs of rejection including widening and blunting of the villi that occurred secondary to inadequate immunosuppression. There appear to be discontinuities in the epithelial cell layer in some areas. (C) Severe rejection is depicted in this specimen with complete loss of the mucosal layer. Consequences of a damaged intestinal mucosal barrier include increased permeability and bacterial translocation.

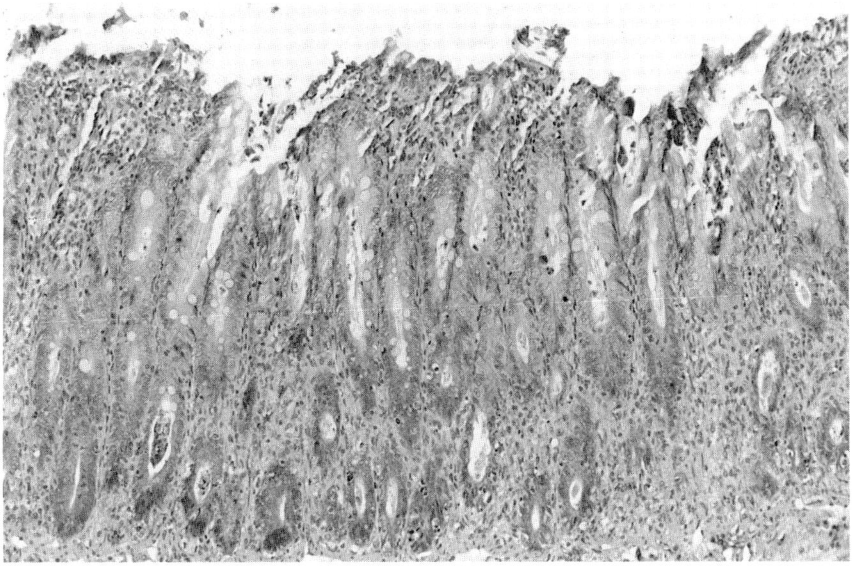

(C)

Fig. 6.2 *continued*

sympathetic and parasympathetic pathways, the small intestine is capable of initiating motor activity. Peristalsis does occur in small intestinal grafts; however, the process may be somewhat less efficient than normal due to the absence of central control and the presence of native intestine anastomosed to the one or both ends of the graft. Abnormal bowel motility may produce stasis of intraluminal contents thereby establishing an environment that is conducive to bacterial overgrowth.[8] Experimental work has revealed that the incidence of barrier failure and subsequent bacterial translocation is increased when bacterial overgrowth is present; therefore, this phenomenon may increase the recipient's incidence of translocation-related systemic infection.[59] The ability of mucus to prevent the attachment of bacteria to enterocytes is well established (see Mucus). Luminal flushing necessary to remove contents from the graft prior to implantation may have an adverse effect on the layer of mucus, therefore, rendering the recipient more susceptible to bacterial translocation and its effects. It is evident that small bowel transplantation has major effects on the mucosal barrier. Whether these effects are clinically relevant and contribute to morbidity and mortality in recipients remain to be demonstrated.

Graft permeability

Utilizing ^{51}Cr-EDTA as a marker, Grant et al. demonstrated increased intestinal permeability in the early postoperative period of rats receiving either isografts or allografts.[71] This finding is probably the result of a variety of factors including ischaemia and would be expected to improve as mucosal regeneration occurs. In the same study, these investigators were able to correlate increased intestinal permeability to ^{51}Cr-EDTA with early graft rejection.[71] This test, in conjunction with endoscopic graft biopsies, was used to assess the first successful small bowel-liver recipient for rejection.[2] In addition to the expected early postoperative increased permeability, the patient experienced an eight-fold increase in urinary excretion of ^{51}Cr-EDTA 9 weeks postoperatively during the only episode of rejection. The values returned to normal following successful treatment of acute rejection. The association of increased small intestinal permeability with early graft rejection enabled the clinician to utilize a simple technique to aid in the early diagnosis of a potentially devastating complication.

Bacterial translocation and the graft

One of the complications of small intestinal barrier failure is bacterial translocation (see Bacterial

Translocation). Although readily demonstrated in the laboratory, the clinical relevance of this phenomenon requires further clarification. Organisms that escape the intestinal lumen and enter the lymphatic system or systemic circulation can probably cause sepsis and other systemic infections; however, the incidence is not known. Endotoxin that crosses the mucosal barrier either by independent translocation or from bacteria already transgressing the barrier has known clinical effects. It contributes to the clinical signs comprising the septic state and probably mediates the multiple system organ failure syndrome.[65]

Although the body of literature providing experimental evidence for bacterial translocation following small bowel transplantation is small, it is convincing and demands the attention of clinicians. Browne et al. studied rats three weeks after orthotopic small bowel transplantation and were able to demonstrate bacterial overgrowth in the transplanted intestine.[72] More importantly, however, they showed that the addition of cyclosporin treatment resulted in translocation of enteric bacterial species to the mesenteric lymph nodes of recipients sacrificed three weeks postoperatively. Fabian and Bollinger demonstrated that bacterial translocation is a rapid process in rats.[73] Seven days after heterotopic small bowel transplantation, they placed kanamycin-resistant *Escherichia coli* into the graft and were able to culture this organism from the mesenteric lymph nodes of the graft as soon as five hours after instillation. Velasco et al. showed that the duration of ischaemia of rat small intestinal isografts placed in the orthotopic position correlated with the incidence of bacterial translocation to the mesenteric lymph nodes, liver, and spleen.[74] These investigators also noted that grafts placed in the heterotopic position did not demonstrate translocation. They postulated that because these grafts were not in continuity with the host's native intestine, bacterial colonization of the donor graft did not occur. Based on these findings, Velasco et al. proposed that exteriorization of the ends of the transplanted graft could serve a role in the early prevention of bacterial translocation. Grant et al. also studied bacterial translocation following small bowel transplantation.[75] In their rat model, the incidence of bacterial translocation was significantly increased during allograft rejection when compared to controls without evidence of rejection.

The association of physical disruption of the mucosal barrier, immunosuppression, and bacterial overgrowth with small bowel transplantation would certainly place recipients at high risk for bacterial translocation and its sequelae.[65] Increased intestinal permeability is indicative of some degree of barrier disruption and has been demonstrated in the immediate postoperative period of both experimental and clinical small bowel transplantation. It is possible that during this period of increased permeability, bacterial translocation is enhanced. At present, graft survival is most dependent on the efficacy of immunosuppressive agents, and small bowel transplantation is no exception. As addressed earlier, bacterial translocation is increased in an environment of impaired immunity; therefore, the recipient of a small bowel graft would be expected to be at risk. The ability of the recipient to mount an immune response to the translocating bacteria would also be impaired by the immunosuppressive agents. The last factor proposed by Deitch to promote bacterial translocation is bacterial overgrowth. Impaired intestinal motility and the use of broad-spectrum antibiotics are known to result in bacterial overgrowth which would be likely to increase the possibility of translocation in intestinal allograft recipients.

Graft barrier enhancement

It is inevitable that mucosal barrier damage occurs during the process of small intestinal transplantation. Methods to fortify the barrier, especially during susceptible periods such as in the immediate postoperative period, need further development. At present, effort must be directed toward limiting barrier damage. Minimizing ischaemic time is an important consideration if mucosal integrity is to be preserved. An aggressive approach should be adopted to monitor small bowel allograft recipients for rejection, and appropriate therapy must be instituted rapidly. Enteral nutrition should be utilized as soon as is feasible to maintain mucosal mass; however, if TPN is required, glutamine-enriched formulas should be employed. The indiscriminate use of broad-spectrum antibiotics and antacids should be avoided to limit bacterial overgrowth.

Conclusion

Transplantation of the small intestine is being performed with increasing frequency in the treatment of short bowel syndrome. This procedure produces unique complications that can disrupt the mucosal barrier and compromise patient outcome. Barrier failure increases intestinal permeability which can lead to bacterial translocation and endotoxemia. The potential clinical consequences of these complications are increased morbidity and mortality; therefore, deliberate effort must be made to minimize damage and expedite recovery of the mucosal barrier.

References

1. Pritchard TJ, Kirkman RL. Small bowel transplantation. *World Journal of Surgery* 1985; **9,** 860–7.
2. Grant D, Wall W, Mimeault R, Zhong R, Ghent C, Garcia B, Stiller C, Duff J. Successful small-bowel/liver transplantation. *Lancet* 1990; **335,** 181–4.
3. Udall JN, Walker WA. Mucosal defence mechanisms. In Marsh MN (ed.) *Immunopathology of the Small Intestine*. Chichester: John Wiley, pp. 3–20, 1987.
4. Schreiber RA, Walker WA. The gastrointestinal barrier: antigen uptake and perinatal immunity. *Ann Allergy* 1988; **61,** 3–12.
5. Chu S-HW, Walker WA. Development of the gastrointestinal mucosal barrier: changes in phospholipid head groups and fatty acid composition of intestinal microvillus membranes from newborn and adult rats. *Ped Res* 1988; **23,** 439–42.
6. Kagnoff MF. Antigen handling by intestinal mucosa: humoral and cell-mediated immunity, tolerance, and genetic control of local immune responses. In Marsh MN (ed.) *Immunopathology of the Small Intestine*. Chichester: John Wiley, pp. 73–102, 1987.
7. Karjalainen J, Martin JM, Knip M, Ilonen J, Robinson BH, Savilahti E, Akerblom HK, Dosch H-M. A bovine albumin peptide as a possible trigger of insulin-dependent diabetes mellitus. *N Engl J Med* 1992; **327,** 302–7.
8. Walker WA. Mechanisms of antigen handling by the gut. *Clin Immunol Allergy* 1982; **2,** 15–40.
9. Jacobson ED. Salivary secretion. In Johnson LR (ed.) *Gastrointestinal Physiology*. St Louis: C V Mosby, pp. 53–62, 1985.
10. Bloch KJ, Bloch DB, Stearns M, Walker WA. Intestinal uptake of macromolecules. VI. Uptake of protein antigen *in vivo* in normal rats infected with *Nippostrongylus brasiliensis* or subjected to mild systemic anaphylaxis. *Gastroenterology* 1979; **77,** 1039–44.
11. Gracey M. Intestinal microflora and bacterial overgrowth in early life. *J Ped Gastroent Nutri* 1982; **1,** 13–22.
12. Nelson DP, Mata LJ. Bacterial flora associated with the human gastrointestinal mucosa. *Gastroenterology* 1970; **58,** 56–61.
13. Drasar BS, Shiner M, McLeod GM. Studies on the intestinal flora. 1. The intestinal flora of the gastrointestinal tract in healthy and achlorhydric persons. *Gastroenterology* 1969; **56,** 71–9.
14. Grand RJ, Watkins JB, Torti FM. Development of the human gastrointestinal tract: a review. *Gastroenterology* 1976; **70,** 790–810.
15. Castro GA. Digestion and absorption. In Johnson LR (ed.) *Gastrointestinal Physiology*. St Louis: C V Mosby, pp. 105–28, 1985.
16. Van Dyke RW. Mechanisms of digestion and absorption of food. In Sleisenger MH, Fordtran JS (eds) *Gastrointestinal Disease: Pathophysiology Diagnosis Management*. Philadelphia: WB Saunders, pp. 1062–88, 1989.
17. Robertson DM, Paganelli R, Dinwiddie R, Levinsky RJ. Milk antigen absorption in the preterm and term neonate. *Arch Dis Children* 1982; **57,** 369–72.
18. Udall JN, Bloch KJ, Vachino G, Feldman P, Walker WA. Development of the gastrointestinal mucosal barrier IV. The effect of inhibition of proteolysis on the uptake of macromolecules by the intestine of the newborn rabbit before and after weaning. *Biol Neonate* 1984; **45,** 289–95.
19. Reilly RW, Kirsner JB. The blind loop syndrome. *Gastroenterology* 1959; **37,** 491–4.
20. King CE, Toskes PP. Small intestine bacterial overgrowth. *Gastroenterology* 1979; **76,** 1035–55.
21. Neutra MR, O'Malley LJ, Secian RD. Regulation of intestinal goblet cell secretion. II. A survey of potential secretagogues. *Am J Physiol* 1982; **242,** G380–7.
22. Walker WA, Abel SN, Wu M, Bloch KJ. Intestinal uptake of macromolecules. V. Comparison of the *in vitro* uptake by rat small intestine of antigen-antibody complexes prepared in antibody or antigen excess. *J Immunol* 1976; **117,** 1028–32.
23. Shub MD, Pang KY, Swann DA, Walker WA. Age related chemical changes in chemical composition and physical properties of mucus glycoproteins from rat small intestine *Biochem J* 1983; **215,** 405–11.
24. Bishop RF, Anderson CM. The bacterial flora of the stomach and small intestine in children with intestinal obstruction. *Arch Dis Childhood* 1960; **35,** 487–91.
25. Kalser MH, Cohen R, Arteaga I, Yawn E, Mayoral L, Hoffert WR, Frazier D. Normal viral and bacterial flora of the human small and large intestine. *N Engl J Med* 1966; **274,** 500–5.
26. Owen RL. Sequential uptake of horseradish peroxidase by lymphoid follicle epithelium of Peyer's patches in the normal unobstructed mouse intes-

tine: an ultrastructural study. *Gastroenterology* 1977; **72,** 440–51.

27. Selby WS, Janossy G, Jewell DP. Immunohistological characterisation of intraepithelial lymphocytes of the human gastrointestinal tract. *Gut* 1981; **22,** 169–76.
28. Dobbins III WD. Human intestinal intraepithelia lymphocytes. *Gut* 1986; **27,** 972–85.
29. Delacroix DL, Hodgson HJF, McPherson A, Dive C, Vaerman JP. Selective transport of polymeric immunoglobulin A in bile. *J Clin Invest* 1982; **70,** 230–41.
30. Perkkiö M, Savilahti E. Time of appearance of immunoglobulin-containing cells in the mucosa of the neonatal intestine. *Ped Res* 1980; **14,** 953–5.
31. Cunningham-Rundles C, Brandeis WE, Good RA, Day NK. Milk precipitins, circulating immune complexes, and IgA deficiency. *Proc Nat Acad Sci USA* 1978; **75,** 3387–9.
32. Lifschitz CH, Shulman RJ. Intestinal permeability tests: are they clinically useful? *J Ped Gastroenter Nutr* 1990; **10,** 283–7.
33. Crissinger KD, Kvietys PR, Granger DN. Pathophysiology of gastrointestinal mucosal permeability. *J Int Med* 1990; **228** (Suppl. 1), 145–54.
34. Porvaznik M. Tight junction disruption and recovery after sublethal γ irradiation. *Rad Res* 1979; **78,** 233–50.
35. Chiu C-J, McArdle AH, Brown R, Scott HJ, Gurd FN. Intestinal mucosal lesion in low-flow states. *Arch Surg* 1970; **101,** 478–83.
36. Cooper BT. Small intestinal permeability in clinical practice. *J Clin Gastroenter* 1984; **6,** 499–501.
37. Cobden I, Dickinson RJ, Rothwell J, Axon ATR. Intestinal permeability assessed by excretion ratios of two molecules: results in coeliac disease. *Br Med J* 1978; **2,** 1060.
38. Cooke WT, Holmes GKT. Gluten-induced enteropathy (celiac disease). In Berk JE, Haubrich WS, Kalser MH, Roth JLA, Schaffner F (eds) *Gastroenterology* Philadelphia, PA: WB Saunders, pp. 1719–57, 1985.
39. Weijers HA, Lindquist B, Anderson CM, Rey J, Schmerling DH, Visakorpi JK, Hadorn B, Gruttner R. Diagnostic criteria in coeliac disease. *Acta Paed Scand* 1970, **59,** 461–4.
40. Menzies IS, Pounder R, Heyer S, Laker MF, Bull J, Wheeler PG, Creamer B. Abnormal intestinal permeability to sugars in villous atrophy. *Lancet* 1979; **2,** 1107–9.
41. Cobden I, Rothwell J, Axon ATR. Intestinal permeability and screening tests for coeliac disease. *Gut* 1980; **21,** 512–18.
42. Ukabam SO, Cooper BT. Small intestinal permeability as an indicator of jejunal mucosal recovery in patients with celiac sprue on a gluten-free diet. *J Clin Gastroenter* 1985; **7,** 232–6.
43. Bjarnason I, Peters TJ, Veall N. A persistent defect in intestinal permeability in coeliac disease demonstrated by a ^{51}Cr-labelled EDTA absorption test. *Lancet* 1983; **1,** 323–5.
44. Fälth-Magnusson K, Jansson G, Stenhammar L, Sundqvist T, Magnusson K-E. Intestinal permeability assessed with different-sized polyethylene glycols in children undergoing small-intestinal biopsy for suspected celiac disease. *Scand J Gastroenterology* 1989; **24,** 40–6.
45. Ukabam SO, Clamp JR, Cooper BT. Abnormal small intestinal permeability to sugars in patients with Crohn's disease of the terminal ileum and colon. *Digestion* 1983; **27,** 70–4.
46. Howden CW, Robertson C, Duncan A, Morris AJ, Russell RI. Comparison of different measurements of intestinal permeability in inflammatory bowel disease. *Am J Gastroenter* 1991; **86,** 1445–9.
47. Magnusson M, Magnusson K-E, Sundqvist T, Denneberg T. Impaired intestinal barrier function measured by differently sized polyethylene glycols in patients with chronic renal failure. *Gut* 1991; **32,** 754–9.
48. Bjarnason I, Smethurst P, Fenn CG, Lee CE, Menzies IS, Levi AJ. Misoprostol reduces indomethacin-induced changes in human small intestinal permeability. *Dig Dis Sci* 1989; **34,** 407–11.
49. Ziegler TR, Smith RJ, O'Dwyer ST, Demling RH, Wilmore DW. Increased intestinal permeability associated with infection in burn patients. *Arch Surg* 1988; **123,** 1313–19.
50. Schrander JJP, Unsalan-Hooyen RWM, Forget PP, Jansen J. [^{51}Cr]EDTA intestinal permeability in children with cow's milk intolerance. *J Ped Gastroenter Nutr* 1990; **10,** 189–92.
51. Edmiston CE, Condon RE. Bacterial translocation. *Surg, Gynecol Obs* 1991; **173,** 73–83.
52. Arnold L, Brody L. Passage of living bacteria through the intact intestinal mucosa. *Proc Soc Exp Biol Med* 1928; **25,** 247–8.
53. Schweinburg FB, Seligman AM, Fine J. Transmural migration of intestinal bacteria: a study based on the use of radioactive *Escherichia coli. N Engl J Med* 1950; **242,** 747–51.
54. Keller R, Engley Jr. FB. Fate of bacteriophage particles introduced into mice by various routes. *Proc Soc Exp Bio Med* 1958; **18,** 577–80.
55. Wells CL, Maddaus MA, Simmons RL. Proposed mechanisms for the translocation of intestinal bacteria. *Rev Infect Dis* 1988; **10,** 958–79.
56. Baker JW, Deitch EA, Li M, Berg RD, Specian RD. Hemorrhagic shock induces bacterial translocation from the gut. *J Trauma* 1988; **28,** 896–906.
57. Deitch EA, Bridges W, Baker J, Ma J-W, Ma L, Grisham MB, Granger DN, Specian RD, Berg R. Hemorrhagic shock-induced bacterial translocation is reduced by xanthine oxidase inhibition or inactivation. *Surgery* 1988; **104,** 191–8.
58. Berg RD. Bacterial translocation from the gastro-

intestinal tracts of mice receiving immunosuppressive chemotherapeutic agents. *Curr Microbiol* 1983; **8,** 285–92.

59. Berg RD. Promotion of the translocation of entric bacteria from the gastrointestinal tracts of mice by oral treatment with penicillin, clindamycin, or metronidazole. *Infection and Immunity* 1981; **33,** 845–61.
60. Alverdy JC, Aoys E, Moss GS. Total parenteral nutrition promotes bacterial translocation from the gut. *Surgery* 1988; **104,** 185–90.
61. Burke DJ, Alverdy JC, Aoys E, Moss GS. Glutamine-supplemented total parenteral nutrition improves gut immune function. *Arch Surg* 1989; **124,** 1396–9.
62. Wells CL, Rotstein OD, Pruett TL, Simmons RL. Intestinal bacteria translocate into experimental intra-abdominal abscesses. *Arch Surg* 1986; **121,** 102–7.
63. Mora EM, Cardona MA, Simmons RL. Enteric bacteria and ingested inert particles translocate to intraperitoneal prosthetic materials. *Arch Surg* 1991; **126,** 157–63.
64. Deitch EA, Berg R, Specian R. Endotoxin promotes the translocation of bacteria from the gut. *Arch Surg* 1987; **122,** 185–90.
65. Deitch EA. The role of intestinal barrier failure and bacterial translocation in the development of systemic infection and multiple organ failure. *Arch Surg* 1990; **125,** 403–4.
66. O'Dwyer ST. Michie HR, Ziegler TR, Revhaug A, Smith RJ, Wilmore DW. A single dose of endotoxin increases intestinal permeability in healthy humans. *Arch Surg* 1988; **123,** 1459–64.
67. Greenman RL, Schein RMH, Martin MA, Wenzel RP, MacIntyre NR, Emmanuel G, Chmel H, Kohler RB, McCarthy M, Plouffe J, Russell JA. A controlled clinical trial of E5 murine monoclonal IgM antibody to endotoxin in the treatment of gram-negative sepsis. *J Amer Med Assn* 1991; **266,** 1097–1102.
68. Ziegler EJ, Fisher CJ, Sprung CL, Straube RC, Sadoff JC, Foulke GE, Wortel CH, Fink MP, Dellinger RP, Teng NNH, Allen IE, Berger HJ, Knatterud GL, LoBuglio AF, Smith CR. Treatment of gram-negative bacteremia and septic shock with HA-1A human monoclonal antibody against endotoxin. *N Engl J Med* 1991; **324,** 429–36.
69. Owens WE, Berg RD. Bacterial translocation from the gastrointestinal tract of athymic (nu/nu) mice. *Infection and Immunity* 1980; **27,** 461–7.
70. Deitch EA. Simple intestinal obstruction causes bacterial translocation in man. *Arch Surg* 1989; **124,** 669–701.
71. Grant D, Lamont D, Zhong R, Garcia B, Wang P, Stiller C, Duff J. ^{51}Cr-EDTA: a marker of early intestinal rejection in the rat. *J Surg Res* 1989; **46,** 507–14.
72. Browne BJ, Johnson CP, Edmiston CE, Hlava MA, Moore GH, Roza AM, Telford GL, Adams MB. Small bowel transplantation promotes bacterial overgrowth and translocation. *J Surg Res* 1991; **51,** 512–17.
73. Fabian MA, Bollinger RR. Rapid translocation of bacteria in small bowel transplantation. *Transplant Proc* 1992; **24,** 1103.
74. Velasco AL, Chung RK, McGowan KL, Steigman CK, Ziegler MM. Bacterial translocation after small intestinal transplantation. *Surg Forum* 1989; **40,** 579–81.
75. Grant D, Hurlbut D, Zhong R, Wang P, Chen H, Garcia B, Behme R, Stiller C, Duff J. Intestinal permeability and bacterial translocation following small bowel transplantation in the rat. *Transplantation* 1991; **52,** 221–4.

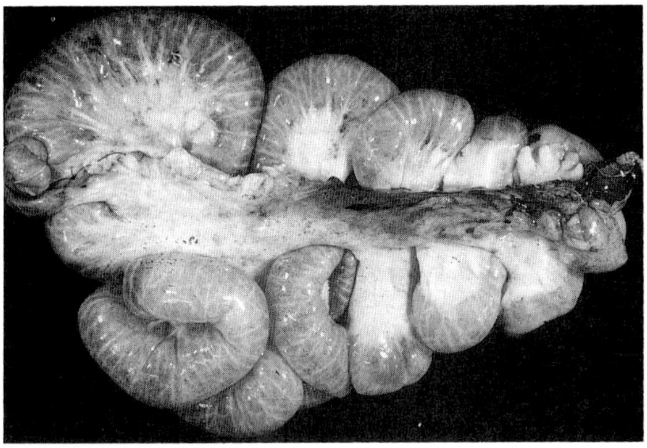

Fig. 7.1 Small intestinal graft harvested from a cadaveric donor. Perfusion, luminal wash-out and storage with Eurocollins solution.

tion. It is well recognized that the rate of postoperative infectious complications increases when the integrity of the gastrointestinal tract is breached.[22] Furthermore, there is extensive literature on gut-mediated sepsis from translocated intraluminal bacteria.[23–5]

Grant et al. have emphasized the important role of the gut as a barrier to bacterial flora. Studies in this laboratory have demonstrated that gut barrier function is lost with preservation injury, leaving the host vulnerable to sepsis from intraluminal microorganisms or toxins.[25,26]

With living-related donors, the gastrointestinal tract can be partially sterilized by an orthograde washout of the luminal content with non-absorbable antibiotics.[27] Experimental studies by Toledo-Pereyra and colleagues demonstrated improved graft survival when antibiotics were added to the luminal perfusate.[28] However, Raju et al. found that using 0.1 per cent kanamycin in the luminal irrigant solution and/or in the preservation solution had no effect on the survival of canine intestinal grafts.[29,30] Park et al. harvested rat intestinal grafts using different combinations of intraluminal and intravascular perfusates and found no differences between the experimental groups.[31] Presently, existing data does not indicate which, if any, intraluminal solutions should be used during retrieval of the small bowel.

Intestinal preservation solutions

Beltzer and Southard have suggested that perfusates and storage solutions should fulfill these conditions for successful organ preservation: (i) reduction of hypothermic-induced cell swelling, (ii) prevention of intracellular acidosis, (iii) enlargement of the interstitial space during the flush-out period, (iv) prevention of tissue injury due to oxygen-free radicals, and (v) regeneration of high-energy phosphate compounds during reperfusion.[32]

Lillehei and co-workers published the first studies on intestinal preservation.[33,34] They showed that perfusion of the vascular bed with an ice-cold saline solution improved mucosal integrity and reduced plasma losses into the abdomen. These studies provided the first description of mucosal oedema with prolonged preservation. In a later experiment, these investigators made the important observations that 1) biopsies taken immediately after revascularization may not accurately reflect the full extent of ischaemic injury to the small bowel and 2) recovery is mandatory to distinguish between early rejection and harvesting damage.[34]

Van Osterhout and associates demonstrated the adverse effect of increasing pressure of the perfusate during intestinal graft harvesting in the rat.[35] A jejunal segment flushed with less pressure (35 cm water) resulted in a viable graft, whereas greater pressure (50–80 cm water) resulted in gangrene. In our own experimental experience, as well in those grafts which were harvested from cadaveric donors (50 cm water),[36,37] varying pressure conditions did not affect graft survival.

Early studies by Toledo-Pereyra and associates found that storage with cryoprecipitated, pooled dog plasma or human plasmanate,[38] and/or the preparation of the intestine with antibiotics, prolonged graft survival in dogs. In later experiments, pulsatile or non-pulsatile flow was used to flush and store the small bowel with pressures of 20–60 mmHg and an average flow of 1–3 ml^{-1} min with good results.[28,39–41]

More recently, two major types of solutions have been used to preserve the small bowel: Collins solution or derivatives, and the University of Wisconsin (UW) solution. To minimize intracellular oedema and potassium loss, Collins-type perfusates have an electrolyte composition which is similar to the intracellular space.[21] The metabolic supply is guaranteed by provision of glucose (Eurocollins). In Eurocollins/Mannitol or Sacks solutions, glucose is replaced by mannitol because glucose permeates only slowly across cell membranes, stimulates cellular anaerobic glycolysis, and augments tissue acidosis.

The UW solution contains raffinose as the carbohydrate source.[32] The roles of the other additives in this solution such as adenosine as an energy source, insulin or steroids as hormones or membrane stabilizers, and allopurinol or glutathione as free radical scavengers – are still poorly defined. However, one thing is clear: UW solution is more effective than Collins solution for the preservation of most solid organs. Modifications of the UW solution that might be advantageous for intestinal harvesting include 1) omitting the adenosine because it could contribute to the formation of oxygen-free radicals, and 2) adding oxygen-radical scavengers such as superoxide dismutase (SOD).[32,42]

Further studies are needed to determine if the solutions for intestinal preservation should contain energy substrates, such as the glucose in Eurocollins or the raffinose in UW solution. Significant protection of the intestinal mucosa occurs when glucose is introduced into the lumen shortly after the onset of ischaemia.[43] Glutamine may also be beneficial in preservation solutions. This substance has been shown to maintain gut morphology and function in a model of intestinal atrophy when given both systemically[44] and intraluminally.[45]

The gut contains high levels of histamine.[46] Histamine dilates intestinal vessels by stimulating vascular H_1 receptors.[47] Histamine also stimulates xanthine-oxidase activity which increases oxygen-free radicals.[48] Data from several sources suggest that histamine release may play an important role in the development of tissue injury during ischaemia and reperfusion. In a syngeneic rat model, systemic plasma histamine concentrations were unchanged 15 minutes after graft reperfusion following harvesting (with UW, hypertonic citrate, or saline solutions), storage up to 48 hours, and transplantation. However, mucosal histamine levels were significantly lower than normal controls.[46] Ackroyd and colleagues have speculated that the local release of histamine results in the oedema, excess mucus secretion, vascular dilatation and engorgement, and finally mucosal haemorrhage that is seen when UW, hypertonic citrate, or saline solutions are used for intestinal preservation.[46]

Taguchi and co-workers have studied the effects of perfusion and storage with Eurocollins solution on smooth muscle function and innervation.[49] If the small bowel was transplanted immediately after harvesting, non-adrenergic inhibition was not impaired. However, there was temporary intrinsic inhibition or partial abolition of the response to acetylcholine and phenylnephrine after perfusion and storage with Eurocollins for 24 hours. Within 8 days these activities were restored, but during this time there was a risk of graft obstruction related to the loss of non-adrenergic inhibition.[50] Storage in Eurocollins solution for 48 hours was unsuccessful.

Scholten[51] and Schweizer[52] have demonstrated that Eurocollins and UW solution are not as effective for intestinal preservation as they are for liver preservation (Table 7.2). In these studies, the best results were achieved using a NaCl-based solution. Most human intestinal recipients have received small bowel grafts that were stored in Eurocollins. There is one report of successful preservation of the human small bowel/liver using 0.9 per cent NaCl containing mannitol (2.1 per cent).[32] There is also one report of severe perfusion injury using UW solution (Fig. 7.2).[37] It may be difficult to perfuse the human small bowel with UW solution because of its high viscosity.

Histological assessment of preservation

Grading systems, which assess small bowel injury due to ischaemia,[31] have been modified to quantitate preservation damage.[52,53] Table 7.2 compares grading systems developed by Chiu,[2] Park,[54] and Schweizer.[52] The latter classification may be the best choice for monitoring clinical grafts as it does not require deep biopsies which could result in perforation or bleeding.[55]

Immediate transplantation with minimal cold ischaemic time has little effect on mucosal integrity.[52,56,57] Figure 7.3 shows an intestinal allograft harvested with Eurocollins from a Lewis rat. This graft was transplanted after 5 hours of cold ischaemia and the biopsy was taken 21 days later. The villi are a normal shape with the exception of a small Gruenhagen's space in the villus tip region. Frödin et al.[56] found that a cold ischaemic time of about 2 hours resulted in graft damage, ranging from Grades 1 to 4. Extension of cold ischaemic time to 18 or more hours resulted in complete destruction of the epithelial layer. A second biopsy, taken 60 minutes after systemic reperfusion, showed increased tissue damage.

Table 7.2 Histological grading of epithelial damage

Grade[1]	Description	Grade[2]	Description	Grade[3]	Description
0	normal mucosa	0	normal mucosa	0	normal mucosa
1	subepithelial Gruenhagen space	1	subepithelial space	1	mild intraepithelial/ subepithelial edema
2	extension of subepithelial spaces	2	extended subepithelial space	2	moderate severe intra-/ subepithelial oedema, beginning epithelial necrosis
3	massive epithelial lifting, villus tip denudation	3	epithelial lifting along villus side		
4	denuded villi exposure of lamina propria	4	denuded villi	3	severe epithelial destruction
5	digestion/disintegration of lamina propria	5	loss of villus tissue		
		6	crypt layer infarction		
		7	transmucosal infarction		
		8	transmural infarction		

[1]Chiu[2], [2]Park[32], [3]Schweizer[54]

Using Sacks solution or a modified histidine buffer (FW solution), tissue injury was evident in the villus, but not in the subepithelial layers, which corresponded to Grade 3 after 5 hours of cold ischaemia.[56] More tissue damage (Grade 4) was observed after a second biopsy was taken 30 minutes after implantation.[56] Graft survival depended on the perfusion solution used: all animals survived in the FW group whereas only 2 of 6 animals survived in the Sacks group. Histological examination of biopsies at 24 hours had a median score of Grade 0.5. Longer preservation times (18 hours) resulted in higher grades of tissue injury and lower survival rates (30 per cent in the FW group; 25 per cent in the Sacks group). Harvesting and storage with normal saline resulted in similar (at 8 hours) or better survival rates (at 10 hours).[52]

Graft histology was characterized by moderate intraepithelial oedema after saline perfusion and moderate subepithelial oedema after UW or Eurocollins flushing. More severe epithelial damage occurred with HTK or St Thomas sol-

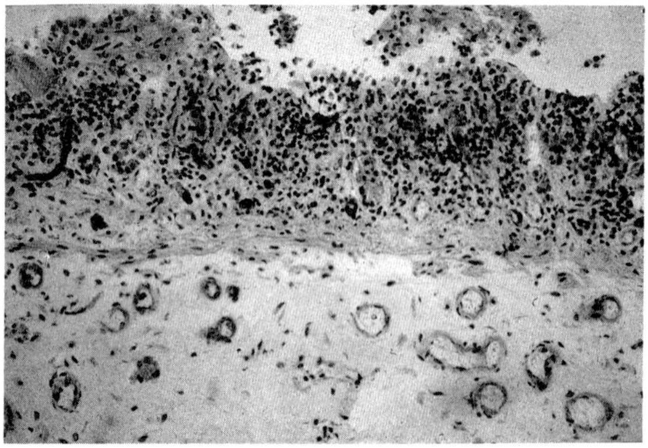

Fig. 7.2 Biopsy from a human intestinal graft taken 2 hours after harvesting with UW solution (CIT 150 min), transplantation and reperfusion with a severe reperfusion injury. Staining against alkaline phosphatase: complete destruction of mucosal structure, no enzyme activity.

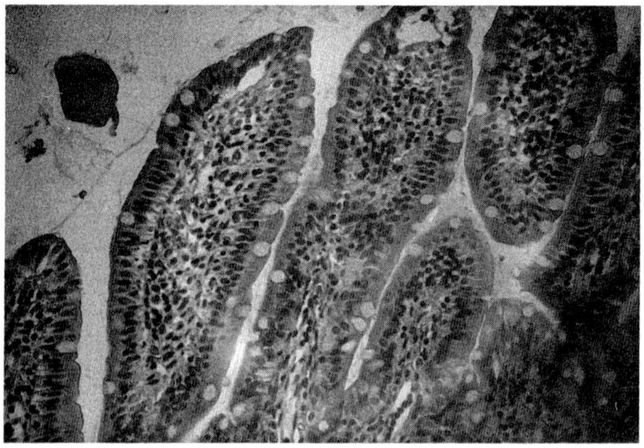

Fig. 7.3 Biopsy taken from a graft of a syngeneic Lewis/ Lewis small bowel transplantation at day 21 postoperative. Graft harvested and stored with Eurocollins, CIT 5 hours. Normal villus shape with small Gruenhagen's space in the villus tip region.

utions. These histological patterns were not reflected in different survival rates because all of the animals survived. With extension of the cold ischaemia time to 5 hours, there were Grade 1 changes with saline, Grade 2 changes with UW and Eurocollins, and Grade 3 changes with HTK and St Thomas. The UW solution provided the best survival rates.[52]

Histological examination of the small bowel graft after implantation does not reliably predict graft or animal survival. After 10 hours of cold ischaemia time, UW-harvested grafts showed mild destruction of the apical part of the villi (Grade 2) but only one animal survived long term, whereas animals with Grade 2 or 3 damage to their grafts, but shorter cold ischaemic times, survived indefinitely.[52] Even when monoclonal antibodies against brush-border enzymes are used, biopsies taken at different preservation times fail to predict subsequent graft function (Schroeder, unpublished results).

An example of reperfusion injury is shown in Fig. 7.2. This biopsy was taken 2 hours after reperfusion of an intestinal allograft, preserved with UW solution, from a cadaveric donor. The section is stained with an antibody directed against alkaline phosphatase. Besides the finding of no enzyme activity, there is also Grade 3 destruction of the epithelium.[52] This graft was removed because of non-function.

Implications for clinical intestinal grafting

The UW solution is probably the best choice for intestinal grafting at the present time. Until the upper limit for safe storage of the human small bowel graft is known, cold ischaemic times should be kept as brief as possible. As there are no markers that reliably predict graft function, it may be advisable to transplant the small bowel in two stages, with heterotopic grafting first and restoration of intestinal continuity at a later time once the graft is known to be working well.

References

1. Raju S, Fujiwara H, Lewin JR, Grogan JB. Twelve-hour and twenty four-hour preservation of small bowel allografts by simple hypothermia. *Transplantation* 1988; **45,** 290–3.
2. Chiu CJ, McArdle AH, Brown R, Scott HJ, Gurd FN. Intestinal mucosal lesion in low-flow states. *Arch Surg* 1970; **101,** 478–83.
3. Brown RA, Chiu CJ, Scott HJ, Gurd FN. Ultrastructural changes in the canine ileal mucosa cell after mesenteric arterial occlusion. *Arch Surg* 1970; **101,** 290–7.
4. Mirkovitch V, Menge H. Movements of water and ions across dog ileal mucosa following ischaemia or occlusion. In Robinson JWL (ed.) *Intestinal Ion Transport.* Lancaster, London, MTP Press, pp. 251–60, 1976.
5. Lundgren O. Studies on blood flow distribution and countercurrent exchange in the small intestine. *Acta Physiol Scand* (Suppl.) 1967; **303,** 1–42.
6. Haglund U, Abe T, Ahren C, Braide I, Lundgren O. The intestinal mucosal lesions in shock. I. Studies on the pathogenesis. *Eur Surg Res* 1976; **8,** 435–447.
7. Svanvik J. Mucosal haemodynamics in the small intestine of the cat during regional sympathetic vaso-constrictor inactivation. *Acta Physiol Scand* 1973; **89,** 19–29.
8. Parks DA, Jacobsen ED. Mesenteric circulation. In Johnson LR (ed.) *Physiology of the Gastrointestinal Tract.* New York, Raven Press, pp. 1649–70, 1987.
9. Fridovich I. The biology of oxygen radicals. *Science* (1978); **201,** 875–80.
10. McCord JM. Free radicals and inflammation: Protection of synovial fluid by superoxide dismutase. *Science* 1974; **185,** 529–31.
11. Batelli MG, Lorenzoni E, Shirpe F. Milk xanthine oxidase type D (dehydrogenase) and type O (oxidase): purification, inter-conversion and some properties. *Biochem J* 1973; **131,** 191–8.
12. Granger DN, McCord JM, Parks DA, Hollworth ME. Xanthine oxidase inhibitors attenuate ischaemia-induced vascular permeability changes in the cat intestine. *Gastroenterology* 1986; **90,** 80–4.
13. Parks DA, Granger DN. Ischaemia-induced vascular changes: Role of xanthine oxidase and hydroxyl radicals. *Am J Physiol* 1983; **245,** G285–9.
14. Bounus G. Role of intestinal contents in the pathophysiology of acute intestinal ischaemia. *Am J Surg* 1967; **114,** 368–75.
15. Bounus G. Acute necrosis of the intestinal mucosa. *Gastroenterology* 1982; **82,** 1457–67.
16. Leaf A. Maintenance of concentration gradients and regulation of cell volume. *Annals NY Academy of Sciences* 1959; **72,** 396–404.
17. Southard JH, Senzig KA, Belzer FO. Effects of hypothermia on canine kidney mitochondria. *Cryobiology* 1980; **17,** 148–53.
18. Burg MA, Orloff J. Active cation transport by kidney tubules at 0°C. *Am J Physiol* 1964; **207,** 983–8.
19. Teichmann R, Stremmel W. Iron uptake by human

small intestine microvillous membrane vesicles. *J Clin Invest* 1990; **86,** 2145–53.
20. Deltz E, Schroeder P, Gebhardt H, Gundlach M, Engemann R, Timmermann W. *Erste Erfolgreiche Dünndarmtransplantation, Chirurg* 1989; **60,** 235–9.
21. Marshall VC, Jablonski P, Scott DF. Renal preservation. In Morris PJ (ed.) *Kidney Transplantation*. Philadelphia, PA, Saunders, pp. 151–82, 1988.
22. Nichols DL. Intra-abdominal sepsis: characterisation and treatment. *J Infect Dis* (Suppl) 1977; **135,** S54.
23. Browne BJ, Johnson CP, Edmiston CE, Hlava MA, Roza A, Telford GL, Adams ME. Small bowel transplantation promotes bacterial overgrowth and translation. *J Surg Res* 1992; **51,** 512–17.
24. Fabian MA, Bollinger RR. Rapid translocation of bacteria in small bowel transplantation. *Transplant Proc* 1992; 241103.
25. Grant DR, Hurlbut D, Zhong R, Wang P, Chen H, Garcia B, Behme R, Stiller C, Duff J. Intestinal permeability and bacterial translocation following small bowel transplantation in the rat. *Transplantation* 1991; **52,** 221–4.
26. Grant DR. Immunosuppression for small bowel transplantation. *Clinical Transplantation* 1991 (special issue); **5,** 563–7.
27. Starzl TE, Todo S, Tzakis A, Alessiani M, Casavilla A, Abu El-magd K, Fung JJ. The many faces of multivisceral transplantation. *Surg Gynecol Obstet* 1991; **172,** 335–44.
28. Toledo-Pereyra LH, Raij L, Simmons RL, Najarian JS. Role of endotoxin and bacteria in long-term survival of preserved small bowel allografts. *Surgery* 1974; **76,** 474–81.
29. Raju S, Didlake RH, Cyirli M, Turner MD, Grogan JB, Achord J. Experimental small bowel transplantation utilising Cyclosporin. *Transplantation* 1984; **38,** 561–6.
30. Shimazu R, Grogan JB, Raju S. Orthotopic non-auxiliary total bowel transplantation using rats: technical procedure. *J Invest Surg* 1988; **1,** 193–200.
31. Park PO, Wallander J, Tufveson G, Haglund U. Cold ischaemic and re-perfusion injury in a model of small bowel transplantation in the rat. *Eur Surg Res* 1991; **23,** 1–829.
32. Belzer FO, Southard JH. Principles of solid-organ preservation by cold storage. *Transplantation* 1988; **45,** 673–6.
33. Lillehei RC, Goott B, Miller FA. The physiological response of the small bowel of the dog to ischaemia including prolonged *in vitro* preservation of the bowel with successful replacement and survival. *Ann Surg* 1959; **150,** 543–60.
34. Eyal Z, Manax WG, Bloch JH, Lillehei RC. Successful *in vitro* preservation of the small bowel, including maintenance of mucosal integrity with chlorpromazine, hypothermia and hyperbaric oxygenation. *Surgery* 1965; **57,** 259–68.
35. Van Oosterhout JMA, de Boer HHM, Jerusalem CR. Small bowel transplantation in the rat: the adverse effect of increased pressure during the flushing procedure of the graft. *J Surg Res* 1984; **36,** 140–6.
36. Schroeder P, Gundlach M, Schweizer E, Deltz E. Small bowel transplantation. *Microsurgery* 1990; **11,** 296–9.
37. Schroeder P, Schweizer E, Deltz E. Clinical small bowel transplantation. *Scand J Gastroent* (Suppl 183) 1991; **26,** I11.
38. Toledo-Pereyra LH, Simmons RL, Najarian JS. Prolonged survival of canine orthotopic small intestinal allografts preservation of 24 hours by hypothermia bloodless perfusion. *Surgery* 1974; **75,** 368–76.
39. Toledo-Pereyra LH. Basic concepts of organ procurement, perfusion and preservation for transplantation. In Toledo-Pereyra LH (ed.) *Organ Procurement*. Academic Press, London, pp. 183–202, 1985.
40. Toledo-Pereyra LH, Najarian JS. Preservatin of the small intestine for allo-transplantation. *Surg Gynecol and Obstet* 1973; **137,** 445–50.
41. Toledo-Pereyra LH, Najarian JS. Small bowel preservation. *Arch Surg* 1973; **107,** 875–7.
42. Luther B, Wolff H, David H, Buchali K, Pahlig G. Die allogene Dünndarmtransplantation – Tierversuche und klinischer Rückblick. *Zentralblatt für Chirurgie* 1987; **112,** 637–52.
43. Chiu CJ, Scott HJ, Fraser NG. II. The protective effect of intraluminal glucose as energy substrate. *Arch Surg* 1970; **101,** 484–8.
44. Schroeder P, Gebhardt H, Brandl M, Wardelmann E, Winkler W, Deltz E. Effect of glutamine-enriched parenteral nutrition on small intestinal glucose and water absorption. *Zeitschrift für Gastroenterologie* 1989; **27,** 300–1.
45. Schweizer E, Elfeldt R, Schroeder P. Glutamine prevents mucosal injury after small bowel transplantation. *Zeitschrift für Gastroenterologie* 1992, in press.
46. Ackroyd EB, Man WK, Simpkin S, Parkin JV, Green CJ. Plasma and mucosal histamine after small bowel transplantation. *Agents and Actions* 1991; **33,** 157–60.
47. Flynn SB, Owen DAA. Histamine receptors in peripheral vascular beds in the cat. *Brit J Pharmacol* 1975; **55,** 181–8.
48. Caty MG, Schmeling DJ, Friedl HP, Oldham KT, Guice KS, Till GO. Histamine: a promotor of xanthine oxidase activity in intestinal ischaemia/re-perfusion. *J Paediat Surg* 1990; **25,** 218–23.
49. Taguchi T, Zorychta E, Sonnino RE, Guttman

FM. Function of smooth muscle and nerve after small intestinal transplantation in the rat: effect of storing donor bowel in Eurocollins. *J Paediat Surg* 1989; **24,** 634–8.

50. Frigo GM, Del Tacca M, Lecchini S. Some observations on the intrinsic nervous mechanism in Hirschprung's disease. *Gut* 1973; **14,** 35–40.
51. Scholten E, Manek G, Green C. A comparison of preservation solutions for long-term storage in rat small bowel transplantation. *Acta Chirurgica Austriaca* 1992; **24,** 5–6.
52. Schweizer E, Gassel A, Deltz E, Schroeder P. Morphological and histological alterations after small bowel transplantation (SBT) – A comparison of different perfusion solutions. *Transplant Proc* 1992; **24,** 1087.
53. Grant D, Wall W, Mimeault R, Zhong R, Ghent C, Garcia B, Stiller C, Duff J. Successful small bowel/liver transplantation. *Lancet* 1990; **335,** 181–4.
54. Park PO, Haglund U, Bulkley GB, Fält K. The sequence of development of intestinal tissue injury after strangulation ischaemia and re-perfusion. *Surgery* 1990; **107,** 574–80.
55. Schroeder P, Schweizer E, Hansmann ML, Hell K, Gundlach M, Gassel J, Deltz E. Monitoring in small bowel transplantation using cytochemistry and immunohistochemistry: a comparison of different techniques. *Transplant Proc* 1991; **23,** 675–6.
56. Frödin L, Bergström C, Haglund U, Park PO, Tufveson G, Wahlberg J. Up to 22-hour preservation of small bowel using transplantation model in the pig. *Transplant Proc* 1990; **22,** 135–6.
57. Fujiwara H, Raju S, Grogan JB, Johnson WW. Organ preservation in small bowel transplantation. *J Invest Surg* 1990; **3,** 23–32.

8

Immunosuppression of small bowel allografts in experimental animals

Stanislaw M Stepkowski and Barry D Kahan

Introduction

More than three decades ago, Lillehei et al.[1] performed successful small bowel autotransplantation in dogs, yet this procedure remains only experimental in humans.[2,3] Among reasons for the delay in implementation are the marked susceptibility to rejection and the unique physiological and bacteriological characteristics of small bowel transplants.[4] One factor contributing to the greater susceptibility is the composite of both host-versus-graft (HVG) and graft-versus-host (GVH) immune responses. Small bowel grafts have the distinctive immunologic characteristic of a large content of immunocompetent cells in the lamina propria, Peyer's patches, and mesenteric lymph nodes (MLN), which mediate GVH reactions.[5] To date, attempts to use drug combinations to offset the rejection problems have not been successful. For instance, initial use of a combination of azathioprine (AZA), steroids, and antilymphocyte serum (ALS) conferred only short prolongation of canine allograft survival compared with untreated controls.[6] Similarly, seven recipients of human small bowel allografts showed rapid rejection using AZA and steroid regimens.[4] The physiological problems that have hindered transplantation in humans include two consequences of organ retrieval: the transection of nerves that regulate bowel peristaltic function and of lymphatic vessels that transport nutrients. Therefore, initially after grafting, the allograft has a severely impaired ability to transport chylomicrons formed in the smooth endoplasmic reticulum of mucosal cells. Thus dietary lipids cannot be delivered into the bloodstream. Similarly, there is retarded transport of long-chain triglycerides into the lymphatics, in contradistinction to short- and medium-chain triglycerides that are readily delivered directly into the portal blood.[7–9] The bacteriological problems stem from post-transplant injury of the intestinal wall, which permits bacterial translocation of luminal contaminants, thereby causing severe infections. The present review addresses progress in the area of immunosuppression to facilitate engraftment, acknowledging that even after this goal is achieved there will be unique physiologic and bacteriologic hurdles.

Donor pretreatment prior to transplantation

Transplants across congeneic rat strain combinations distinguished mild versus lethal GVH which was induced by Class I versus Class II major histocompatibility (MHC) barriers, respectively. A Class I MHC disparity induced only erythema and dermatitis, producing death in only 2 in 10 animals at 30 days post-grafting. All other hosts recovered and survived more than 100 days. In contrast, transplants across a Class II MHC disparity uniformly induced acute lethal GVH disease.[10] The large quantity of lymphoid tissue engrafted with small bowel transplants is responsible for its induction.[11] Transplantation of vascularized MLN alone without the intestinal component produced lethal GVH.[12] The disease was abrogated by mesenteric lymphadenectomy of small bowel grafts.[13] Two approaches have been used to reduce the load of lymphoid tissue in small bowel grafts: namely, shortening the length of the transplanted intestine, and pretreating the donor to decrease the lymphoid content of the graft.[14,15]

Irradiation of donor small bowel prevented the development of GVH, but accelerated the rejection (HVG) of the allografts.[16] Untreated WAG (RT-1^u) allografts were rejected by Brown Norway (BN; RT-1^n) recipients at 16.6 ± 2.6 days with 35 per cent of the animals showing GVH symptoms. Grafts irradiated with 10 or 5 gray (Gy) were rejected at 7.5 ± 0.9 days or 11.5 ± 0.4 days, respectively. The adverse effect of higher radiation doses may be due to reduction of graft lymphatic elements facilitating the access of recipient cells to produce rejection. Radiation-induced damage to the mucosa, which facilitates bacterial translocation, may be mitigated by shielding the intestinal component of the allograft while treating the MLN.[16]

Another method of donor pretreatment is the administration of massive doses of ALS, in order to deplete T cells from MLN.[17] Grafts from Lewis (LEW; RT-1^l) rats that had been pretreated for 48 hours prior to transplantation displayed indefinite survival in (LEW × BN) F_1 recipients. Contrariwise, untreated animals succumbed at 15.7 ± 2.8 days. Pretreatment with ALS for only 4 hours was ineffective. Furthermore, polyclonal ALS was more effective than R73 mouse monoclonal antibody directed against the rat α/β T cell receptor, which after a 48-hour course only prolonged recipient survival to 34.4 ± 24.9 days. The difference between the results obtained after ALS versus R73 antibody treatment may be related to the ability of the polyclonal, but not monoclonal, antibodies to avidly bind complement, thereby lysing lymphocytes.

Although reduction in lymphoid mass is useful, ablation is not helpful. Subclinical GVH appears to be beneficial to small bowel allograft acceptance.[18] PVG (RT-1^c) transplants caused fatal GVH disease in (PVG × DA) F_1 recipients within 21 days, but DA (RT-1^a) grafts survived 30 days with only mild GVH symptoms. Mesenteric lymphadenectomy of the PVG donors increased the survival of small bowel grafts by only a few days, whereas lymphadenectomy of DA-donor allografts produced indefinite transplant survival free of GVH. Thus, in the settings of mild to moderate GVHD, a reduced quantity of lymphoid tissue may induce tolerance.[18]

Cyclosporin immunosuppression for small bowel transplantation

The advent of cyclosporin (CsA) sparked renewed interest in small bowel transplantation, an endeavour that had been quiescent following the numerous failures observed using AZA-based regimens. CsA inhibits T cell proliferation and differentiation by blocking transcription of early activation genes, including those encoding cytokines such as interleukin-2 (IL-2).[19] Prodrug CsA binds to a family of 17 kDa proteins denoted cyclophilins, cis-trans peptidyl-prolyl isomerases, which in turn forms a quaternary complex of calcineurins A and B, Ca^{2+}, and calmodulin. This complex formation inhibits the catalytic action of calcineurin, an intermediate step in the calcium-dependent T cell receptor signalling pathway from the cell membrane to the nucleus.[20,21] Several studies have demonstrated that CsA prolongs the survival of orthotopic and heterotopic small bowel transplants in rats,[22–29] pigs,[30–32] dogs,[33–35] and primates.[36] In rat models, the effectiveness of CsA strongly depends upon the degree of donor-recipient histoincompatibility and the degree of host immunoresponsiveness. Low CsA doses (5 mg/kg) delivered subcutaneously (s.c.) to LEW recipients for 14 days produced both indefinite survival of orthotopic BN small bowel allografts[22] and donor-specific unresponsiveness, as evidenced by delayed rejection of challenge BN, but not third-party ACI, skin allografts (Table 8.1). A 14-day continuous intravenous (i.v.) infusion of 4 or 8 mg/kg CsA by osmotic pump prolonged the survival of heterotopic BN allografts in LEW recipients from 12.5 ± 2.2 days to 21.6 ± 6.3 or 31.0 ± 1.8 days, respectively[23] (Table 8.2). An increased 15 mg/kg CsA dose also produced long-term graft survival, but caused opportunistic infections leading to a 60 per cent mortality within 100 days with gram-negative bacteria, which translocated from gut lumen to MLN and other organs.[24] The mortality rate was 60 per cent in the 15 mg/kg and 85 per cent in the 24 mg/kg CsA dose groups. In contrast, only 2 out of 10 LEW untreated hosts of a syngeneic LEW graft displayed translocation. Both native and transplanted mesenteric lymph nodes of CsA-treated animals showed translocation of bacteria with progressive sepsis due to *Escherichia coli (E. coli)* and *Staphylococci* in the liver, spleen, and lungs.[24] Thus, bacterial translocation may represent the outcome of impaired defence mechanisms of immunosuppressed hosts as well as compromised mucosal integrity caused by rejection. CsA completely inhibited the capacity of hosts to mount a mucosal immune response of anti-cholera toxin IgA antibodies.[25] Interestingly, overimmunosuppression was prevented by switching the daily intramuscular (i.m.) treatment course with 15 mg/kg CsA to an alternate-day regimen from day 6 to 28, resulting in long-term BN graft survival in LEW recipients[26,27] (Table 8.1) with neither HVG nor GVH within 8 months post-grafting.

The 28-day course of 15 mg/kg CsA produced variable responses, depending upon the dosage and the donor/recipient combination. BN small bowel allografts survived indefinitely in LEW recipients.[25] Contrariwise, ACI (RT-1^a) transplants were rejected at 130.3 ± 66.1 days with histological evidence of chronic rejection and symptoms of GVH disease with mononuclear infiltration around the bile ducts and patchy proliferative responses in the spleen.[26] Similarly, orthotopic 20 cm and 40 cm jejunal Buffalo (BUF; Rt-1^b) allografts in LEW recipients treated i.m. with 5 mg/kg CsA for 28 days were rejected at 58.2 ± 13.7 days and 129 ± 7.4 days, respectively.[28] Thus, the survival times of neither ACI- nor BUF-allografts were as prolonged as those of BN transplants in LEW hosts.

Administration of high (25 mg/kg) CsA doses delivered i.m. for 14 days prolonged the survival of orthotopic WAG (RT-1^u) transplants in BN recipients to 42.5 ± 2.7 days.[29] Addition of maintenance CsA 15 mg/kg doses on alternate days thereafter indefinitely extended survival to 100 days in only 7 out of 30 animals. Most long-term allograft recipients displayed GVH disease, suggesting that CsA immunotherapy produces less inhibition of the GVH response. Furthermore,

Table 8.1 CsA effect on orthotopic small bowel allograft survival in rats

Donor	Recipients	CsA therapy mg/kg	Days	Rate	Survival MST±SD	Authors
BN	LEW	—	—	—	10±0	Shimazu, et al.[22]
BN	LEW	5	14	s.c.	>100	Shimazu, et al.[22]
BN	LEW	15	14	s.c.	>100	Shimazu, et al.[22]
BN	LEW	5	14	s.c.	>100	Shimazu, et al.[22]
(BNx LEW)Fi	LEW	15	28	i.m.	>360	Langrehr, et al.[27]
BN	LEW	15	28	i.m.	>100	Lee and Schraur[26]
BUF	LEW	—	—	—	—	Kimuta, et al.[28]
BUF (20 cm)	LEW	5	28	i.m.	58.2±13.7	Kimuta, et al.[28]
BUF (40 cm)	LEW	5	28	i.m.	129.1±7.4	Kimuta, et al.[28]
ACI	LEW	—	—	—	7.2±0.7	Langrehr, et al.[27]
ACI	LEW	15	5	i.m.	30.3±13	Langrehr, et al.[27]
ACI	LEW	15	28	i.m.	130±66.1	Langrehr, et al.[27]
WAG	BN	—	—	—	16.6±2.7	Saat, et al.[29]
WAG	BN	25	6	i.m.	38.3±3.8	Saat, et al.[29]
WAG	BN	25	14	i.m.	42.5±2.7	Saat, et al.[29]

Table 8.2 CsA effect on heterotopic small bowel allograft survival in rats

Donor	Recipients	CsA therapy mg/kg	Days	Rate	Survival MST±SD	Authors
BN	LEW	—	—	—	12.5±2.2	Stepkowski, et al.[23]
BN	LEW	4	14	i.v.	21.6±6.3	Stepkowski, et al.[23]
BN	LEW	8	14	i.v.	31.0±1.8	Stepkowski, et al.[23]

the regimen was less effective across the WAG-to-BN disparity than the ACI- or BUF-to-LEW combinations.

In spite of these favourable results in rats, immunosuppressive therapies have failed to achieve long-term small bowel allograft survival in large animals. Triple-combination therapy with AZA/prednisolone/ALS was ineffective in both dogs[6] and humans.[4] CsA produced much better results,[2] particularly in the porcine model. While untreated pigs rejected small bowel allografts in 11.3 ± 3.2 days, hosts receiving a 21-day course of 15 mg/kg CsA i.v. combined with steroids, followed by oral gavage of tapering doses of CsA beginning at 30 mg/kg, uniformly displayed prolonged allograft survival (121 ± 3.2 days). Increased i.v. CsA doses of 20 mg/kg led to fatal pneumonitis. Autopsies of the small bowel grafts failed to show acute or chronic rejection or GVH disease during the period of CsA treatment.[30] Rejection occurred only when CsA was discontinued at 100 days post-grafting, although 7 of 6 recipients maintained satisfactory nutrition and weight gain without continued immunosuppression.

CsA (10 mg/kg) i.m. prolonged short, segmental, jejunal porcine allograft survivals to 80.9 ± 22.3 days.[31] Three animals survived 16 months, although 8 pigs died between 12 and 136 days of complications caused by venous obstruction, abdominal abscesses, or grafts rejection. The 5 animals that survived at least 90 days without complications displayed mean whole blood CsA trough levels of 372 ± 158 ng/ml. Although short segmental allografts probably are less antigenic than full-length transplants, they may not provide a sufficient absorptive surface, particularly for vitamin B_{12}.

Oral rather than i.m. or i.v. administration of CsA (30 mg/kg) was ineffective: all animals rejected their allografts within 10 to 53 days. However, in a triple-drug combination with AZA (50 mg/day) and prednisolone (40 mg/day), oral CsA (15 mg/kg) produced long-term survival of orthotopic porcine allografts (60 days) without rejection.[32] Systemic sepsis or localized intra-abdominal abscesses occurred in 5 out of 30 recipients. The nature of the benefit conferred by combination immunosuppressive therapy is unclear, since the studies did not establish the amount of CsA alone that was necessary to achieve a similar effect as the triple combination.

Small bowel transplants in dogs present an even greater challenge than pig hosts to tailor a CsA-based immunosuppressive protocol.[31–35] A regimen of CsA (25 mg/kg) given one day prior to and daily after surgery was potentiated by prednisolone (200 mg/day for two days followed by 5 mg/day) plus AZA (2 mg/kg) daily thereafter. The 52.2 ± 14-day survival of hosts treated with the triple combination was significantly longer than the 9.2 ± 0.9 days survival of untreated controls. However, histological examination of the allografts in the combination-treatment group showed graft damage, including shortening of the villi, dilatation of lacteals, widening of the interstitial space, and necrosis accompanied by severe cellular infiltration.[33] Other therapeutic protocols were even less successful. For instance, *ex vivo* irradiation (10 Gy) of the donor small bowel graft did not improve its survival. Addition of donor pretreatment with ALS[34] failed to further prolong the survival of short segmental jejunal grafts (110 cm) that had undergone mesenteric lymphadenectomy prior to transplantation into hosts treated with CsA (16 mg/kg) i.v. and prednisolone (10 mg/day). These allografts showed a lymphoplasmacytic infiltration of nerves, vessels, and submucosal tissues.[35] Thus, neither CsA alone, nor CsA-prednisolone or CsA-AZA-prednisolone combinations, overcomes small bowel allograft rejection in the mongrel canine model.

In rhesus monkey primates,[36] allografts irradiated with 1.5 Gy and then transplanted into hosts treated with CsA (40 mg/kg), solumedrol (2 mg/kg), and AZA (5 mg/day) showed survival in 3 out of 4 instances without microscopic evidence of rejection. After an average time of 75.3 days, opportunistic bacterial infection necessitated euthanasia.[36]

Thus, the effect of pharmacologic agents on small bowel allograft survival primarily depends on the species and, secondarily, on the histoincompatibility barrier. In the CsA-susceptible rat, a short course of CsA induced indefinite survival of BN grafts in LEW hosts, but was ineffective across the WAG-to-BN combination. Although relatively low CsA doses combined with prednisolone maintained good small bowel graft function in pigs, even CsA-based triple therapy was ineffective in dogs. The efficacy of overly aggressive immunosuppressive regimens was limited by opportunistic infections.

Table 8.4 RAPA effect on heterotopic small bowel allograft survival in rats

Donor	Recipient	RAPA Treatment mg/kg	Days	Route	Survival (days)	Authors
BUF	WFu	—	—	—	10.5±0.5	Stepkowski, et al.[23,60]
BUF	WFu	0.8	14	i.v.	25±4.6	Stepkowski, et al.[23,60]
BN	LEW	—	—	—	12.5±2.5	Stepkowski, et al.[23,60]
BN	LEW	0.8	14	i.v.	21.6±2.0	Stepkowski, et al.[23,60]
BN	LEW	1.6	14	i.v.	26.5±2.8	Stepkowski, et al.[23,60]
LEW	(BNxLEW)F_1	—	—	i.v.	12.3±2.8	Stepkowski, et al.[23,60]
LEW	(BNxLEW)F_1	0.8	14	i.v.	21.2±5.2	Stepkowski, et al.[23,60]
(BNxLEW)F_1	LEW	—	—	—	12.2±3.6	Stepkowski, et al.[23,60]
(BNxLEW)F_1	LEW	0.8	14	i.v.	40.8±5.6	Stepkowski, et al.[23,60]

Table 8.5 RAPA and RAPA/CsA effect on orthotopic small bowel allograft survival in rats

Donor	Recipient	Treatment RAPA mg/kg	RAPA Days	CsA mg/kg	CsA Days	Survival (days) MST±SD	Authors
BN	LEW	—	—	—	—	10.2±2.0	Wang, et al.[61]
BN	LEW	0.08	14	—	—	11.2±2.7	Wang, et al.[61]
BN	LEW	—	—	4	14	8.8±0.4	Wang, et al.[61]
BN	LEW	0.08	14	4	14	32.6±5.1	Wang, et al.[61]
BN	LEW	0.2	14	—	—	14.6±3.2	Chen, et al.[62]
BN	LEW	0.8	14	—	—	36±10.8	Chen, et al.[62]
BN	LEW	—	—	2	14	16.4±2.4	Chen, et al.[62]
BN	LEW	0.2	14	2	14	36.8±7.9	Chen, et al.[62]

showed that RAPA synergistically acts with CsA to block T cell responses to alloantigens. Subtherapeutic amounts of RAPA (0.01 mg/kg) and CsA (0.5 mg/kg) prolonged BUF heart survival in WFu recipients to 20.8 ± 2.7 days ($p < 0.001$). A combined course of RAPA (0.04 mg/kg) with CsA (2 mg/kg) prolonged heart allograft survival to 93.4 ± 23.9 days ($p < 0.001$), as compared with 14.2 ± 4.9 days or 14.2 ± 9.9 days for RAPA or CsA alone, respectively. A similar strategy was tested in small bowel transplantation.[62] Individually, neither RAPA (0.08 mg/kg) nor CsA (4 mg/kg) protected orthotopic BN allografts from rejection by LEW recipients, but the two-drug combination prolonged survival to 32.6 ± 5.1 days (P< 10.001; Table 8.5). Similar results were obtained using other RAPA and CsA doses.[62] Orthotopic small bowel allograft survival was prolonged to 14.6 ± 3.2 days and 36.0 ± 10.8 by a 14-day course of RAPA at 0.2 and 0.8 mg/kg, respectively. CsA (2 mg/kg) alone prolonged allografts to 16.4 ± 2.4 days. The combination of RAPA (0.02 mg/kg)/CsA (2 mg/kg) extended recipient survival to 36.8 ± 7.9 days. Thus, the combination of RAPA and CsA seems to proffer the most potent immunosuppressive regiment available for small bowel allotransplantation.

Conclusions

Successful small bowel transplantation depends upon the development of immunosuppressive regimens capable of inhibiting both GVH and HVG immune responses without enhancing the infectious complications. Experiments in rats documented that the efficacy of immunosuppressive agents varies widely. They are ineffective in some strain combinations, yet induce donor-specific tolerance in other combinations. Similar findings emerged in large animal models. Although sufficient immunosuppression was difficult to achieve in dogs, long-term small bowel allograft survival was readily obtained in pigs. Further experimental work must concentrate on developing new agents and on testing combination drug regimens in order to achieve effective immunosuppression without toxic effects. Small bowel transplantation is a particular target for tolerance induction protocols in view of the unique physiological susceptibility and bacteriologic hazards of this organ.

Acknowledgements

The authors wish to thank Dawn Trejo for typing the manuscript and tables, and B. Lee Ligon, M A, for editing and preparing the manuscript.

References

1. Lillehei RC, Goot B, Miller FA. The physiologic response of the small bowel of the dog to ischemia including prolonged in vitro preservation of the bowel with successful replacement and survival. *Ann Surg* 1959; **150,** 543–59.
2. Grant D. Intestinal Transplantation: Current Status. *Transplant Proc* 1989; **21,** 2869–71.
3. Wood RFM. International symposium on small bowel transplantation. *Transplant Proc* 1990; **22,** 2423–6.
4. Fortner JG, Sichuk G, Litwin SD, Beattie EJ. Immunological responses to an intestinal allograft with HL-A identical donor-recipient. *Transplantation* 1972; **14,** 531–5.
5. Monchick GJ, Russell PS. Transplantation of small bowel in the rat. Technical and Immunological Consideration. *Surgery* 1971; **70,** 693.
6. Hardy MA, Quint Y, Stale D. Effect of antilymphocyte serum and other immunosuppressive agents on canine jejunal allografts. *Ann Surg* 1970; **171,** 51–60.
7. Alfin-Slater RB. Lipids. In Aftergood L (ed.) *Modern Nutrition in Health and Disease.* Philadelphia, PA, Lea and Febiger, pp. 113–41, 1980.
8. Senior JR. The place of medium chain triglycerides. *Am J Med Sci* 1969; **257,** 75–80.
9. Kocandrle V, Houttiun E, Prohaska JV. Regeneration of the lymphatics after autotransplantation and hemotransplantation of the entire small intestine. *Surg Gynecol Obstet* 1966; **122,** 587–92.
10. Lück R, Klempnauer J, Steiniger B. Genetic requirements for the development of graft-versus-host rejection following small bowel transplantation. *Transplant Proc* 1990; **22,** 2529–30.
11. Jamieson NV, Joysey V, Friend PJ, Marcus R, Ramsbottom S, Johnston PS, Williams R, Calne RY. Graft-versus-host disease in solid organ transplantation. *Transplant Intern* 1991; **4,** 67–71.
12. Lück R, Klempnauer J, Steiniger B. Transplantation of MHC incompatible vascularized mesenteric lymph nodes: identical pattern of lethal graft-versus-host disease as induced by small bowel grafts. *Transplant Proc* 1990; **22,** 2332.
13. Lück R, Klempnauer J, Steiniger B. Abrogation of lethal graft-versus-host disease in MHC disparate small bowel transplantation in the rat by mesenteric lymphadenectomy. *Transplant Proc* 1990; **22,** 2471.
14. Starzl MJ, Moynihan HL, Lee KKW, Schrout WH. Rejection of ileal versus jejunal allografts. *Transplantation* 1989; **47,** 424–7.
15. Freeman JS, Chamberlain EC, Reemtsma K, Steinmuller D. Prolongation of rat heart allografts by donor pretreatment with immunosuppressive agents. *Transplant Proc* 1971; **3,** 580–2.
16. Saat RE, deBruin RWF, Heineman E, Jackel J, Marquet RL. Irradiation of the donor combined with cyclosporine treatment of the recipient prevents graft-versus-host disease and leads to prolonged survival of small-bowel allografts. *Transplant Proc* 1990; **22,** 2465–6.
17. Shaffer D, Ubhi CS, Simpson MA, Gottschalk R, Milford EL, Maki T, Monaco AP. Prevention of graft-versus-host disease following small bowel transplantation with polyclonal and monoclonal antilymphocyte serum. *Transplantation* 1991; **52,** 948–52.
18. Clark CLI, Price BA, Malcolm P, Lear PA, Wood RFM. Graft-versus-host disease in small bowel transplantation. *Br J Surg* 1991; **78,** 1077–9.
19. Hess AD. Effect of cyclosporine A on the immune response: pivotal role of the interleukin-2/interleukin-2 receptor autocrine pathway. In Thomson AW (ed.) *Cyclosporine: Mode of Action and Clinical Application.* Boston/London: Dordecht, pp. 24–33, 1989.
20. Schrieber SL, Liu J, Albers MW, Karmacharya R, Koh E, Martin RK, Rosen MK, Standaert RF, Wandless TJ. Immunophilin-ligand complexes as probes of intracellular signaling pathways. *Transplant Proc* 1991; **23,** 2839–44.
21. Thomson SQ, Duncan JI. The influence of cyclosporine A on T-cell activation, cytokine gene expression and cell mediated immunity. In Thomson AW (ed.) *Cyclosporine: Mode of Action and Clinical Application.* Boston/London: Dordecht, pp. 50–81, 1989.
22. Shimazu R, Grogan JB, Raju S. Long term survival

of orthotopic bowel allografts in the rat treated with short-term low-dose cyclosporine. *Transplantation* 1988; **4,** 673–7.
23. Stepkowski SM, Chen H, Wang M, Daloze P, Kahan BD. Inhibition of host-versus-graft and graft-versus-host responses after small bowel transplantation in rats by rapamycin. *Transplantation* 1992; **53,** 258–64.
24. Browne BJ, Johnson CP, Edmistors CE, Hlava MA, Moore GH, Roza AM, Telford G, Adams MB. Small bowel transplantation promotes bacterial overgrowth and translocation. *J Surg Res* 1991; **51,** 512–17.
25. Xia W, Kinkman RL. Inhibitory effect of cyclosporine on specific secretory IgA production against cholera toxin in small bowel transplantation. *Transplant Proc* 1991; **23,** 682–3.
26. Lee KKW, Schraut WH. Structure and function of orthotopic small bowel allografts in rats treated with cyclosporine. *Am J Surg* 1986; **151,** 55–60.
27. Langrehr JM, Lee KKW, Wachs ME, Lee TK, Starzl MJ, Venkataramanan R, Kunz HW. Comparison of the effectiveness of cyclosporine A in small-bowel transplantation using different rat strain combinations. *Transplant Proc* 1990; **22,** 2533–5.
28. Kimura K, La Rosa C, Money SR, Jaffe B. Segmental intestine transplantation in rats with resected entire small bowel, ileocecal valve on cecum. *J Surg Res* 1988; **45,** 349–56.
29. Saat RE, deBruin RWF, Heineman E, Jeekel J, Marquet RL. The limited efficacy of cyclosporine in preventing rejection and graft-versus-host disease in orthotopic small bowel transplantation in rats. *Transplantation* 1990; **50,** 347–77.
30. Grant D, Duff, J, Zhong R, Garcia B, Lipohar C, Keown P, Stiller C. Successful intestinal transplantation in pigs treated with cyclosporine. *Transplantation* 1988; **45,** 279–84.
31. Kimura K, LaRosa CA, Blank MA, Jaffe B. Successful segmental intestinal transplantation in enterectomized pigs. *Ann Surg* 1989; **121,** 158–64.
32. Kaneko H, Hancock W, Schweizer RT. Progress in experimental porcine small-bowel transplantation. *Arch Surg* 1989; **124,** 587–92.
33. Fujiwara H, Grogan JB, Raju S. Total orthotopic small bowel transplantation with cyclosporine. *Transplantation* 1987; **44,** 469–73.
34. Shimazu R, Raji S, Fujiwara H, Grogan JB. Experimental small bowel transplantation: alternative strategies for graft prolongation. *Transplant Proc* 1985; **24,** 1253–7.
35. Banner B, Dean P, Williams J. Morphologic features of rejection in long-surviving canine small bowel transplants. *Transplantation* 1988; **46,** 665–9.
36. Thale D, Waldorf KA, Kleinschmidt J, Pearl R, Seyfer AE. Small intestine transplantation in nonhuman primates. *J Pediatr Surg* 1991; **26,** 914–20.
37. Dumont F, Staruch MJ, Koprak SL, Melino MR, Sigal NH. Distinct mechanisms of suppression of murine T-cell activation by the related macrolides FK 506 and Rapamycin. *J Immunol* 1990; **144,** 251–8.
38. Siekierka JJ, Staruch MJ, Hung SHY, Sigal NH. FK 506, a potent novel immunosuppressive agent, binds to a cytosolic protein which is distinct from the cyclosporine binding protein, cyclophilin. *J Immunol* 1989; **143,** 1580–3.
39. Liu J, Farmer JD, Lane WS, Friedman J, Weissman I, Schrieber SL. Calcineurin is a common target of cyclophilin-cyclosporine A and FKBP-FK 506 complexes. *Cell* 1991; **66,** 807–15.
40. Schreiber SL, Crabtree GR. The mechanism of action of cyclosporine A and FK 506. *Immunol Today* 1992; **13,** 136–42.
41. Ochiai T, Nakaijma K, Nagota M, Suzuki T, Asano T, Uematsu T, Goto T, Hori S, Kenmochi T, Nakagoori T, Isono K. Effect of a new immunosuppressive agent, FK 506, on heterotopic cardiac allotransplantation in the rat. *Transplant Proc* 1987; **19,** 1284–6.
42. Todo S, Demetris AJ, Ueda, Imventarza O, Okuda K, Casavila A, Cemaj S, Chatab A, Mazzaferro V, Rhoe BS, Tonghua Y, Makowka L, Starzl TE. Canine kidney transplantation with FK 506 alone or in combination with cyclosporine and steroids. *Transplant Proc* 1987 (Suppl. 6); **19,** 57–61.
43. Todo S, Ueda, Demetris AJ, Imventarza O, Nalasnik M, Vankataramanan R, Makowka L, Starzl TE. Immunosuppression of canine, monkey, and baboon allografts by FK 506: with special reference to synergism with other drugs and tolerance induction. *Surgery* 1988; **104,** 239–49.
44. Rodo S, Demetris A, Ueda Y, Imventarza O, Cadoff E, Zeevi A, Starzl TE. Renal transplantation in baboons under FK 506. *Surgery* 1989; **106,** 444–51.
45. Starzl TE, Todo S, Fung J, Demetris AJ, Vankataramanan R, Jain A. FK 506 for human liver, kidney, and pancreas transplantation. *Lancet* 1989; **2,** 1000–3.
46. Langrehr JM, Hoffman KA, Miller AR, Lee KKW, Demetris AJ, Schraut WH. Indefinite small bowel allograft survival after limited immunosuppression therapy is not due to specific hyporesponsiveness. *Transplant Proc* 1991; **23,** 3248–50.
47. Murase N, Demetris AJ, Matsuzaki T, Yagihashi A, Todo S, Fung J, Starzl TE. Long survival in rats after multivisceral versus isolated small-bowel allotransplantation under FK 506. *Surgery* 1991; **110,** 87–98.
48. Takeda Y, Okajima K, Iga C, Date K, Ryo T, Niki M, Asaka K, Tezuka T, Isozaki H. Effect of

FK 506 on the survival of rat small bowel allografts. *Transplant Proc* 1991; **23,** 3251.
49. Hoffman AL, Makowka L, Banner B, Cai X, Cramer DV, Pascualone A, Todo S, Starzl TE. The use of FK 506 for small bowel intestine allotransplantation. Inhibition of acute rejection and prevention of fatal graft-versus-host disease. *Transplantation* 1990; **49,** 483–90.
50. Santiago SF, Fukuzawa M, Azuma T, Okada A. Effect of donor pretreatment with FK 506 upon small intestine allotransplantation in rats. *Transplant Proc* 1991; **23,** 3243–5.
51. Fukuzawa N, Santiago S, Nakata S, Shirakura, Okada A. Effect of donor-specific transfusion and FK 506 on small intestine allotransplantation. *Transplant Proc* 1991; **23,** 3252–4.
52. de Bruin RWF, Hogen Esch H, Heineman E, Jeekel J, Marquet RL. Fulminant graft-versus-host disease after FK 506 treatment in fully allogeneic small bowel transplantation. *Transplant Proc* 1991; **23,** 3257–9.
53. Yoshimi F, Nakamura K, Zhu T, Suzuki M, Funakoshi T, Carrieri G, Wu T, Furukawa H, Demetris AJ, Todo S, Starzl TE. Canin total orthotopic small bowel transplantation under FK 506. *Transplant Proc* 1991; **23,** 3240–2.
54. Vezina C, Kudelski A, Sehgal SN. Rapamycin (AY-22, 989), a new antifungal antibiotic: I taxonomy of the producing spteptomycete and isolation of the active principle. *J Antibiot (Tokyo)* 1975; **28,** 721.
55. Bierer BE, Mattila PS, Standaert RF, Herzenberg AL, Burakoff SJ, Crabtree G, Schreiber SL. Two distinct signal transmission pathways in T lymphocytes are inhibited by complexes formed between immunophilin and either FK 506 or rapamycin. *Proc Natl Acad Sci USA* 1990; **87,** 9231–5.
56. Metcalf SM, Richards FM. Cyclosporine, FK 506, and rapamycin: some effects on early activation events in serum-free, mitogen-stimulation mouse spleen cells. *Transplantation* 1990; **49,** 798–802.
57. Kahan BD, Gibbons S, Tajpa N, Stepkowski SM, Chou T. Synergistic interactions of cyclosporine and rapamycin to inhibit immune performances of normal human peripheral blood lymphocytes *in vitro*. *Transplantation* 1991; **51,** 252–39.
58. Calne RY, Lim S, Samaan A, Collier SJ, Pollard SG, White DJG. Rapamycin for immunosuppression in organ allografting [Letter]. *Lancet* 1989; **2,** 227–8.
59. Stepkowski SM, Chen H, Daloze P, Kahan BD. Rapamycin, a potent immunosuppressive drug for vascularized heart, kidney, and small bowel transplantation in the rat. *Transplantation* 1991; **51,** 22–6.
60. Stepkowski SM, Kahan BD. Rapamycin and cyclosporine synergistically prolong heart and kidney allograft survival. *Transplant Proc* 1991; **23,** 3262–4.
61. Wang M, Stepkowski SM, Kahan BD. Synergistic interaction of rapamycin and cyclosporine on orthotopic small bowel allograft survival in rats. (In preparation.)
62. Chen H, Wu J, Xu D, Aboujaoude M, Stepkowski SM, Kahan BD, Daloze P. The effect of rapamycin on orthotopic small bowel transplantation in the rat. *Transplant Proc* 1992; **24,** 1157–8.

Donor and graft irradiation

The increased sensitivity of lymphocytes to various forms of irradiation relative to other cell types has long been known.[23] It is not surprising then that many attempts have been made to decrease the lymphocyte content of allografts using irradiation protocols with the aim of decreasing graft immunogenicity.

In the rat model, both heart[24] and kidney[25] grafts can be significantly prolonged with whole body irradiation (WBI) of the donor prior to transplantation. However, in an early study using a canine renal allograft model,[26] Hume et al. were unsuccessful in prolonging graft survival with up to 1500 rad WBI of the donor 24 hours preoperatively with no recipient immunosuppression. One possible explanation of the failure of Hume's experiment is the finding that 1200 rad WBI applied to the donor at 96 hours prior to transplant significantly prolonged kidney graft survival and was associated with profound donor lymphopenia, whereas the same dose of irradiation given at 72 hours preoperatively failed to have a significant effect on either the peripheral lymphocyte count or allograft survival.[25] Since WBI of the donor is not clinically applicable, attention has been focused on irradiation of the isolated allograft itself.

Irradiation of isolated heart and kidney allografts was also shown to significantly prolong survival in several rat strain combinations,[27] although with high-responder strains massive doses were required. The mechanisms underlying the beneficial effect of irradiation, as well as other pretreatment regimens, on prolonging graft survival were elucidated by McKenzie et al.[28,29] who were the first to quantify the effect of the donor pretreatment regimen on the interstitial dendritic cell population and correlate this with histological examination of the graft as well as measurement of graft survival. They found that only after depletion of more than 95 per cent of the interstitial dendritic cell population in the rat cardiac and kidney models was graft survival significantly prolonged. They further showed that MHC Class I antigen expression was not altered by the graft pretreatment protocols. The explanation for the failure of many graft pretreatment regimens most likely lies in the fact that a small number of residual dendritic cells within the graft can still lead to sufficient recipient immunity and graft rejection.

With the small bowel, attempts to modify the graft have often been less successful owing to the much greater number of passenger leukocytes which not only induce a very strong rejection reaction from the host but are capable of causing GVHD. Although the depletion of passenger leukocytes would theoretically decrease both rejection of the graft and GVH reactions, it is well known that GVHD in itself confers a general immunosuppressive effect[30] and a partial, controlled GVH reaction may in fact be advantageous. An attempt to balance the rejection and GVH reactions must be made. From the experience with other organs complete depletion of passenger leukocytes in a small intestinal graft will be extremely difficult if not impossible to achieve. However, any decrease in graft immunogenicity would favour graft acceptance and presents no detrimental effect to the recipient. In the (Lewis × Brown Norway)F_1 hybrid to Lewis rat unidirectional rejection model, Monchik and Russell[3] found that 700 rad WBI of the small bowel donors 4 to 24 hours before transplantation allowed indefinite survival of heterotopic small bowel allografts compared to a mean graft survival of only 8.9 days in untreated controls. In the unidirectional GVHD rat combination (Lewis to $LBNF_1$), *ex vivo* irradiation of small intestinal grafts with 1000 rad immediately before transplant was found to completely prevent GVHD in heterotopic auxiliary and orthotopic models.[31] Lower doses of irradiation had no significant effect. They also showed that these grafts were functionally normal with no evidence of radiation injury up to 6 months postoperatively.

In fully-allogeneic models of small bowel transplantation in the rat the effects of irradiation of the allograft are more equivocal. In a low-responder strain combination (Lewis-ACI) graft irradiation has been shown to significantly prolong small bowel allograft survival.[32] This effect, although statistically significant, was not dramatic, with a mean survival time of approximately 12 days. In combinations where the rejection response is stronger, irradiation of the donor or small bowel graft has not been shown to prolong graft survival.[33,34] These authors propose that the small bowel may contain a relatively large number of antigen-presenting cells (APC) which are radioresistant and facilitate rejection even with near total depletion of other graft passenger leukocytes.

GVHD can also be eliminated with WBI of the

donor in fully-allogeneic rat combinations.[35] In the WAG ($RT1^u$) to BN ($RT1^n$) combination, untreated recipients of orthotopic small bowel grafts died of rejection after approximately 16 days. When WAG donors were treated with 10 Gy WBI (1 gray,Gy = 100 rad) on the day of transplantation, GVHD was eliminated. However, the mean survival time was actually decreased significantly compared to controls. It was proposed that the lack of GVHD-induced immunosuppression led to an accelerated rejection response, which was confirmed histologically.[36] Additional studies combined donor WBI with recipient cyclosporin immunosuppression in this same strain combination. Although GVHD was eliminated after donor irradiation, mean survival time (MST) was not significantly increased compared with recipient immunosuppression with cyclosporin alone.[37] In fully-allogeneic small bowel transplant models, which are more applicable clinically, the critical balance between rejection and GVHD becomes more apparent.

With total orthotopic small bowel transplants in fully-allogeneic dogs the effects of graft irradiation are also variable. Cohen et al.[2] found that untreated controls had a MST of approximately 9 days with GVHD as the most likely cause of death. When isolated small bowel grafts from these dogs were irradiated with 150 rad immediately prior to transplantation, survival times were again approximately 9 days. However, this group had typical pathologic changes of rejection at autopsy. No GVHD was seen in this group. When a decreased dose of irradiation was applied (50 rad) to the graft, the MST was significantly prolonged to 28 days. With this protocol it appeared that a favourable balance between GVHD and rejection had been achieved. Higher doses of graft irradiation, up to 250 rad, resulted in the early death of all recipients secondary to graft necrosis. On the other hand, Williams et al.[38] found that up to 1500 rad irradiation applied to canine small bowel grafts *ex vivo* was well tolerated with no detectable radiation injury for up to 2 years following transplantation. In fact, when technical deaths were excluded, recipients receiving grafts irradiated with 750 rad as well as chronic cyclosporin immunosuppression survived >200 days on average. There were no histologic signs of GVHD in these recipients. Cyclosporin absorption was not impaired in recipients of grafts treated with up to 1500 rad measured through 13 weeks postoperatively. The majority of these recipients did have sublethal acute rejection although less severe than normally expected. When 1500 rad *ex vivo* irradiation was used, rejection was decreased and no GVHD was evident. Unfortunately this was associated with an increased incidence of infection which decreased survival times significantly compared with the 750 rad group.

In an outbred pig model of total orthotopic intestinal transplantation,[39] graft irradiation combined with recipient immunosuppression using cyclosporin did not prolong graft survival when compared to cyclosporin alone. With doses of 500 cGy there were no significant differences between irradiated bowel and non-irradiated controls with respect to cyclosporin absorption, triglyceride absorption, glucose absorption, faecal fat measurements, serum albumin, total protein and haemoglobin levels or postoperative body weight. There was also no detectable radiation damage evident at autopsy up to one year post-transplantation.

A major disadvantage of graft irradiation is the possibility of architectural or functional damage of the graft. The pathological features of radiation enteropathy have been well described: mucosal atrophy, ulceration and cellular abnormalities; submucosal oedema and hyalinosis; focal hyalinization and fibrosis of the muscularis propria; serosal thickening with vascular ectasia; obliterative angiitis with thrombosis; strictures; fistulae; and frank infarction secondary to major vascular occlusion.[40–3] With the dosages used in the previously discussed protocols, the incidence of significant radiation injury should be low. Under ischaemic conditions, as with *ex vivo* irradiation, rat small bowel can withstand up to 1050 rad irradiation without subsequent injury.[44] Human lymphocytes are slightly more radiosensitive *in vitro* with almost all dying within two days following irradiation with 900 rad.[45,46] However, adequate studies regarding the functional consequences of small intestinal irradiation are difficult to conduct in view of the total denervation and lymphatic interruption which occurs with small bowel transplantation and causes additional functional impairment.

Another more basic concern, referred to earlier, is the possibility that the antigen-presenting cells most responsible for induction of the rejection response, i.e. dendritic cells, are not as radiosensitive as lymphoid cells within the graft. Thus, even with the production of significant lymphopenia after donor WBI or with significant inactivation of these cells following *ex vivo* irradiation of the isolated graft, the APC may still be in sufficient numbers to elicit a sufficient immunologic reaction for graft destruction. This point is illustrated by the recent finding that the proliferative response of canine and human mesenteric lymph node lymphocytes to phytohemagglutinin and their response in an MLC are inhibited in a dose-dependent fashion by irradiation of the small bowel allograft.[47] With 1500 rad approximately 90 per cent inhibition is seen. However, transplantation of this irradiated human allograft resulted in severe acute rejection necessitating graft removal 14 days postoperatively. Klinkert et al.[48] found that dendritic cells from a number of rat tissues were the predominant accessory cells capable of antigen presentation and found that metabolic activity was required for these cells to function in this capacity. However these cells were radioresistant with continued function after treatment with 1000 rad gamma irradiation.

Ultraviolet irradiation

The effects of direct ultraviolet (UV) irradiation (272–400 nm spectrum) on graft immunogenicity have been studied mainly in pancreatic islet transplant models. Lau and Hardy et al. found that direct UV irradiation of islets (900 J/m^2) allowed indefinite survival in both allograft and xenograft models with normal endocrine function, although this was partially strain dependent.[49–51] These islet allografts were also cultured for 24 hours prior to transplantation and the authors state that UV irradiated islets not cultured are rejected in an unmodified manner. In parallel *in vitro* experiments, the capacity of isolated rat dendritic cells to act as stimulators in MLC with allogeneic responders was completely eliminated when exposed to 900 J/m^2 UV-B (280–320 nm) irradiation. In contrast, gamma irradiation did not affect the stimulatory capacity of these isolated dendritic cells. The effect of UV irradiation is not through the physical elimination of Ia-positive dendritic cells, but rather through metabolic inactivation, although the exact mechanism is unknown.[52] Although these experiments clearly show that UV irradiation decreases allostimulation and even xenostimulation, the applicability of this method of allograft pretreatment is limited and with larger solid organ grafts the extent of graft passenger cell depletion may be insufficient to have a significant effect.

Lymphocytotoxic drug pretreatment

It is not surprising that the earliest attempts at donor or graft pretreatment involved the use of relatively non-specific cytotoxic and cytolytic agents, given the predominant role of these agents in clinical transplantation. Cyclophosphamide, methylprednisolone, methotrexate and more recently cyclosporin have been studied extensively. Guttman and Lindquist first showed prolongation of kidney allografts in a rat model after the donor was pretreated with a multidrug combination including cyclophosphamide, procarbazine, and methotrexate.[53] Similar pretreatment protocols also had a beneficial effect in rat heart allografts.[54] Additional experiments showed passenger leukocytes to be the drug-sensitive cell population affected. In subsequent studies involving donor and allograft pretreatment in canine renal transplantation conflicting results were obtained with the majority of data showing no prolongation of graft survival.[55–7] Differing preservation and graft perfusion protocols probably accounted for some of the variability in these results. In the 1970s, several clinical studies were conducted examining the effect of donor pretreatment with cyclophosphamide and methylprednisolone in cadaveric kidney transplantation. Despite encouraging results indicating decreased severity of rejection and improved overall graft survival,[58–9] subsequent studies provided equivocal results[60–3] and these trials were eventually abandoned.

As with other treatment regimens involving the donor or allograft, the most likely clinically applicable beneficial effect will be achieved when combined with recipient immunosuppression possibly at a decreased level. Kahn et al.[64] recently demonstrated significantly prolonged survival of rat heart allografts with a combination of donor pretreatment with a single injection of methotrexate and a variety of recipient immunosuppressive protocols compared with either treatment alone. They achieved a 60 per cent increase in graft survival by this combined treatment protocol.

Experience with donor or allograft pretreatment with immunosuppressive agents in small bowel transplantation is limited. In a highly histoincompatible rat small bowel allograft model

(DA-Lewis), donor pretreatment with FK 506 has been shown to significantly prolong small bowel allograft survival when combined with recipient treatment with a sub-therapeutic dosing regimen of FK 506.[65] Reduction of recipient immunosuppression in this study resulted in a significantly decreased rate of infection. Donor pretreatment with FK 506 was not effective when used without recipient immunosuppression. In the same rat strain combination, however, donor pretreatment with cyclosporin was ineffective in prolonging graft survival even when combined with low-dose cyclosporin immunosuppression of the recipient.[66]

Because routine immunosuppression of the recipient has failed to completely eliminate the rejection response, these donor pretreatment regimens should not be abandoned but rather studied in well-designed, randomized studies.[67] In future experiments the effect of pretreatment regimens must be correlated with a quantitative measurement of donor organ passenger leukocytes and carried out under more controlled conditions. Newer, more selective lymphocytotoxic agents may prove more effective when used in pretreatment regimens.

Mesenteric lymphadenectomy

Direct physical manipulation of the small bowel graft has also been attempted in an effort to decrease its immunogenicity. In the rat, the surgical removal of mesenteric lymph nodes from small bowel grafts has been clearly shown to eliminate graft-versus-host disease in the unidirectional GVHD model (Lewis to $LBNF_1$).[68] Recipients of Lewis small bowel allografts pretreated with mesenteric lymphadenectomy (MLE) were comparable to isografted control animals with normal weight gain postoperatively and mean survival times >300 days.[69] The importance of immunocompetent lymphocytes within the mesenteric lymph nodes (MLN) in eliciting GVHD was also documented by injecting isolated MLN lymphocytes intraperitoneally and causing a lethal GVHD identical in timing and severity to that caused by total small bowel transplantation. Others have documented that immunocompetent cells in the MLN of the graft are more important in causing GVHD than lymphocytes in other compartments of the small bowel graft.

The effect of MLE in rejection and fully-allogeneic models in which both GVHD and rejection can occur is less clear. In a fully-allogeneic rat model using heterotopic SBT, grafts treated with MLE actually had increased rejection when compared to those grafts untreated prior to transplantation.[70] The elimination of a graft-versus-host reaction after MLE, which is known to be immunosuppressive, may have led to the increase in graft rejection seen in this study.

Although very effective in unidirectional GVHD rat models, another potential disadvantage with this pretreatment regimen is the possible functional disturbance secondary to the interruption of the mesenteric lymphatic system which may lead to absorption deficiencies. While MLE is an excellent tool for studying the GVH reaction after small bowel transplantation, clinical application of this technique appears limited.

Antilymphocyte serum pretreatment

Polyclonal antilymphocytic serum (ALS) when given *in vivo* induces profound peripheral blood and tissue lymphopenia with depletion of circulating T lymphocytes from the paracortical area of peripheral lymph nodes.[71,72] Because of these properties, ALS was also one of the initial agents used in donor or graft pretreatment protocols in which the goal is to decrease passenger leukocytes in the transplanted organ.

Donor pretreatment with ALS was shown to be effective in prolonging the survival of rat kidney[73] and heart allografts.[24] However, attempts to correlate the effect on graft survival with donor lymphopenia were unsuccessful. Longer surviving grafts were often from donors with the least degree of lymphopenia and vice versa. Oluwole and associates subsequently confirmed the effectiveness of ALS donor pretreatment given 24 hours before harvest of the graft in the rat heart allograft model.[74] They also used Indium-111 oxine-labelled leukocytes to show that ALS pretreatment was associated with an approximate 25 per cent depletion of graft lymphocytes. Callender et al. showed ALS graft perfusion to be effective when combined with low-dose azathioprine recipient immunosuppression[75] in canine renal allografts.

Several studies conducted in our laboratory have shown that donor pretreatment with ALS is a very effective modality in preventing GVHD following SBT. Shaffer et al. totally eliminated GVHD in a unidirectional rat GVHD model when the donors were pretreated on day -2 and -1 relative to transplant with polyclonal rabbit anti-rat ALS at a dose of 5 ml/kg/day via either intraperitoneal or intravenous routes.[76] A single dose of ALS eliminated GVHD if given at least 48 hours prior to small bowel graft harvest. Graft function was examined in detail and found to be normal in the recipients of pretreated grafts compared to isografted controls. Polyclonal ALS proved more effective than donor pretreatment with a pan-T cell monoclonal antibody (R73) given in several different treatment schedules. The effectiveness of ALS in preventing GVHD also correlated well with profound lymphopenia in the peripheral blood and in the graft MLN. Monoclonal antibody pretreatment induced peripheral blood lymphopenia but failed to deplete lymphocytes from the MLN which have been shown to be an important source of cells inducing the GVH reaction. In other studies, *ex vivo* perfusion of the small bowel graft with ALS was ineffective in preventing GVHD in the same model.[77] The role of complement activation after ALS treatment *ex vivo* needs to be studied in a more detailed manner in future experiments.

Donor pretreatment with ALS in a similar regimen eliminated GVHD in a fully-allogeneic model of SBT (BN-Lewis) and when combined with cyclosporin immunosuppression there was indefinite survival of all recipients.[78] In recipients treated with cyclosporin alone, sublethal GVHD occurs 4 to 6 weeks postoperatively with significant weight loss and other classic symptoms of GVHD. This study also documented the importance of treatment with ALS at least 48 hours before organ harvest. In a similar study, goat anti-rat antilymphocyte globulin (ALG) given to the small bowel donor prolonged survival when recipients were treated with a very low-dose cyclosporine regimen.[79] Reduction in recipient immunosuppression is obviously a goal of any donor pretreatment regimen.

In the first successful combined small bowel/liver transplant in humans, GVHD developed in the recipient despite donor pretreatment with Minnesota ALG.[5] Fortunately this GVHD episode was transient and clinically mild and may have been attenuated by the ALG treatment. It has to be recognized that in the clinical situation only a very limited time is available for donor pretreatment with ALS.

Monoclonal antibody – immunotoxin perfusion protocols

For a cell to function as an antigen-presenting cell several requirements must be met. One requirement is the expression of MHC Class II antigen (Ia antigen) on the cell surface. The other essential property is the ability to form a complex with its cell surface MHC antigen and the foreign or alloantigen (i.e. antigen processing).[80] Many attempts have been made at decreasing the immunogenicity of grafts prior to transplantation by either the elimination or inactivation of I-region associated (Ia) antigen positive (MHC Class II) stimulatory cells within the graft by perfusion with monoclonal antibodies (MAb) and immunotoxins aimed at the Ia antigen itself. Ia antigens play a crucial role in a variety of immunologic responses including T lymphocyte-macrophage interactions, recognition of foreign or alloantigen, and interaction of T and B lymphocytes in antibody production.[81]

Schwartz et al. showed that anti-Ia antisera, but not anti-H-2K or anti-H-2D (Class I) antibodies, inhibited T lymphocyte proliferative responses to a variety of antigens *in vitro*.[82] T lymphocyte subpopulations have different susceptibilities to anti-Ia antisera and complement. The lytic effects of anti-Ia serum have been shown in some studies to be directed against antigen-specific T cells and not accessory cells, e.g. macrophages and non-antigen specific T cells, *in vitro*.[83] This study also reported that primed T-helper cells and T cells which proliferate in response to alloantigen in the MLR are completely resistant to lysis by anti-Ia serum and complement. Other *in vitro* studies have shown that the inhibition of T cell proliferation in response to certain antigens may in fact be secondary to the action of anti-Ia serum against Ia positive macrophages which act as antigen-presenting cells.[84] The percentage of antigen-presenting macrophages actually lysed with anti-Ia antiserum and complement is fairly low. However, remaining macrophages are unable to act as APC possibly because of a very low density of Ia antigen on their cell surface.[85]

Pretreatment of allografts with anti-Ia monoclonal antibodies has been effective in several transplant models. Faustman et al.[86] demonstrated markedly prolonged survival of mouse allogeneic islets of Langerhans without recipient immunosuppression after pretreatment with a specific anti-Ia monoclonal antibody and complement. Islet cells are known to lack I region gene products,[87] therefore anti-Ia serum treatment apparently removes Ia positive passenger lymphoid cells important in rejection initiation. Islet allograft acceptance is promptly terminated by injection of donor splenocytes into established transplant recipients, demonstrating the importance of donor antigen-presenting passenger cells in causing rejection. Modest prolongation of whole pancreas allograft survival after pretreatment in this manner has also been confirmed in a rat model.[88] In preliminary studies, murine atrial allografts transplanted beneath the kidney capsule of recipients pretreated with anti-Ia serum and complement were also found to have significantly decreased rejection when examined histologically 21 days post-transplantation.[89] Canine renal allograft survival has also been prolonged with this method.[90] Sone et al. reported significantly prolonged rat cardiac allograft survival with donor heart perfusion with anti-Ia monoclonal antibody although this was limited, with rejection occurring by 45 days post-transplant.[81] When murine bone marrow allografts were perfused *ex vivo* with anti-T cell MAb GVHD was completely eliminated; however the rejection response was increased reciprocally.[91] Only after treatment of both donor and recipient to deplete T cells was long-term survival achieved. In a more recent study, simultaneous T cell and accessory cell depletion with the antilymphocyte/antimonocyte monoclonal antibody K31 and complement was shown to strongly decrease the immunogenicity of bone marrow grafts as measured by the decreased accessory and allostimulatory capacities *in vitro*.[92] These responses were restored with the addition of autologous peripheral adherent cells but not with autologous T cells, showing the importance of accessory cells for the allostimulatory response of human bone marrow grafts. Bone marrow pretreatment regimens with immunotoxins are now in clinical trials and may be effective in GVHD prophylaxis.[93] The effect of this treatment on bone marrow engraftment and late rejection is not as completely studied.

Ex vivo perfusion of canine liver allografts with OKIal MAb (anti-MHC Class II) also significantly decreases early acute rejection following orthotopic liver transplant.[94] The ability of sinusoidal lining cells, which are known to express Class II antigens, to stimulate allogeneic lymphocytes *in vitro* was also decreased in the perfused liver group compared with non-perfused controls.

More recently, masking of MHC Class I antigen molecules on the grafted tissue with F(ab′)2 antibody fragments prior to transplantation has been shown to effectively prevent rejection of xenogeneic islets of Langerhans in a human to BALB/c mouse model.[95] This regimen is based on the theory that destruction of target cells by cytotoxic T lymphocytes requires the presence of MHC Class I antigen on the cell surface.

The uncertainty in the potency of monoclonal antibodies (MAb) has led to the idea of conjugating these to cytotoxic agents, forming immunotoxins. A number of proteins, e.g. ricin, abrin and diphtheria toxin, are able to act as cytotoxins but have very non-specific actions involving nearly all cell types. By conjugating these to MAb specific targets can be affected. Nakahara et al., using a mouse anti-Ia MAb conjugated with ricin A chain (immunotoxin 13.4) directed against I-E^k antigens, showed specific elimination of stimulatory spleen cells in a murine MLR.[96] Further studies also showed inhibition of the MLR in rats after pretreating stimulatory cells with this immunotoxin.

With small bowel allografts the abundance of Ia positive lymphoid cells in the Peyer's patches and mesenteric lymph nodes as well as Ia expression of intestinal epithelial cells makes this pretreatment regimen more difficult. The intestinal mucosa is also very susceptible to ischaemic injury; hypersecretion, hypermotility and low vascular resistance are all potential pitfalls in graft perfusion. *In situ* perfusion via cannulae introduced transhepatically into the portal vein and through the aorta distal to the superior mesenteric artery allowed for normothermic perfusion of the small bowel graft with a pharmacologically modified perfusate for three hours without excessive graft injury in a rat model.[97] Mucosal damage was seen histologically before transplant, but had recovered by the seventh postoperative day in full-thickness biopsies with no permanent ischaemic mucosal damage. Various attempts have been made to deplete T cell subsets and accessory passenger cells from the small bowel with equivocal results. Very modest prolongation of survival following orthotopic small bowel transplantation in the Lewis to DA rat model after perfusion with a combination of MAb directed against MHC Class II antigen, macrophages and dendritic cells has been observed.[98] Incomplete antigen-presenting cell depletion was probably responsible for the limited improvement seen.

In a unidirectional GVHD model in the rat,

Shaffer et al.[99] demonstrated that generalized depletion of T lymphocytes by MAb pretreatment of donor animals significantly prolonged survival by decreasing the GVH response, with some animals surviving indefinitely. However, selective depletion of CD4 or CD8 positive T cell subpopulations had no effect on the development of GVHD. That either T cell subset can mediate lethal GVHD has also been shown in several murine bone marrow transplant models.[91,100] Ingham Clark et al. have also shown significantly prolonged survival of heterotopic small bowel allografts perfused with a pan-T cell MAb (OX19)-ricin conjugate in a unidirectional GVHD model.[101] However, all recipients eventually died secondary to severe GVHD less than two months after transplantation. In subsequent studies it has been shown that penetrance of this immunotoxin into the paracortex of the mesenteric lymph node and the T cell areas of the Peyer's patches is very low.[102] This most likely explains the limited beneficial effect in decreasing GVHD following small bowel transplantation. However, this method of donor pretreatment remains very attractive and requires further study. As mentioned earlier, the effects of GVHD elimination by these treatment protocols must be studied in the fully-allogeneic model to determine the effect on rejection of the allograft before determining applicability to the clinical situation.

Clinical considerations

Donor or allograft modification has the theoretical advantage of reducing graft immunogenicity and the subsequent risks of chronic recipient immunosuppression. However, several basic issues need to be clarified prior to successful clinical application.

One controversial issue concerns the ability of host antigen-presenting cells to present graft alloantigen to its own effector cells and lead to graft destruction, even if effective graft antigen-presenting cell depletion has been achieved. Evidence that host APC, with different MHC type, cannot present alloantigen and that graft rejection requires the presence of APC with donor-type MHC antigen is provided by Lechler and Batchelor.[13] They found that the addition of recipient strain APC to APC-depleted grafts did not restore the allostimulatory response whereas addition of very small numbers of donor strain APC promptly led to rejection. Others support the idea that host APC do present alloantigen, although in a less efficient manner.[10]

Another issue is the ability of other graft cells to act as APC after the more classic APC have been depleted.[103] There is substantial evidence that endothelial cells in humans express Class II MHC antigen[104] and under certain conditions can present alloantigen and stimulate the host immune response.[105,106] These studies have documented that isolated endothelial cells can act as APC in mixed lymphocyte-endothelium culture *in vitro*. These issues have obvious implications for the effectiveness of pretreatment protocols aimed at depleting graft passenger stimulatory cells.

Another important issue with more immediate clinical relevance is whether attempts to eliminate the GVH reaction following small bowel transplantation are necessary to the success of such grafts.[107] It is now well known that following small bowel transplantation there is a large bidirectional transfer of lymphoid cells between the graft and the recipient. This results in the near replacement of graft lymphoreticular cells with recipient type cells. Iwaki et al. found that after 10 to 12 weeks postoperatively, this lymphoid repopulation was complete.[108] Simultaneously, graft lymphoid cells migrate to lymphoid tissues in the recipient, creating 'local chimerism'.[109] This cell trafficking usually occurs in the absence of rejection and GVHD under adequate immunosuppression. It has been suggested that with the newer immunosuppressive agents now available (e.g. FK 506) the risk of GVHD in clinical small bowel transplantation is minimal. It has further been suggested that any attempt at donor modification is unnecessary because of these immunosuppressive drugs.

Under both cyclosporin and FK 506 immunosuppression following clinical small bowel transplantation, donor lymphoid cells have been consistently detected in the recipient.[5,108] As mentioned earlier, in most cases this has not led to clinically significant GVHD. However, in several cases there has been significant GVHD which on one occasion led to the death of the recipient.[109] In experimental small bowel transplantation it has also been shown that donor cells remain in the graft on a long-term basis, thereby prolonging at least the theoretical risk of GVHD.[110]

Although these issues remain unresolved, the basic philosophy underlying pretreatment of the donor organ with the aim of reducing its immunogenicity remains valid. A reduction of graft immunogenicity may lead to improved allograft survival and/or a reduction in deleterious effects of chronic immunosuppression. Donor pretreatment should be viewed as an adjunct to the newer, more selective and more potent immunosuppressive agents as well as more specific and effective monoclonal antibody therapy.

References

1. Kirkman RL, Lear PA, Madara JL, Tilney NL. Small intestine transplantation in the rat – immunology and function. *Surgery* 1984; **96,** 280–6.
2. Cohen Z, MacGregor AB, Moore KTH, Falk RE, Langer B, Cullen JB. Canine small bowel transplantation. *Arch Surg* 1976; **111,** 248–53.
3. Monchik GJ, Russell PS. Transplantation of small bowel in the rat: Technical and immunological considerations. *Surgery* 1971; **70**, 693–702.
4. Lillehei RC, Goot B, Miller FA. Homografts of the small bowel. *Surg Forum* 1959; **10,** 197–201.
5. Grant D, Ware W, Mimeault R, Zhong R, Ghent C, Garcia B, Stiller C, Duff J. Successful small bowel/liver transplantation. *Lancet* 1990; **335,** 181–4.
6. Starzl TE, Rowe MI, Todo S et al. Transplantation of multiple abdominal viscera. *JAMA* 1989; **261,** 1449–57.
7. Williams JS, Sankary HN, Foster PF, Lowe J, Goldman GM. Splanchnic transplantation: an approach to the infant dependent on parenteral nutrition who develops irreversible liver disease. *JAMA* 1989; **261,** 1458–62.
8. Hardy MA, Chabot J, Tannenbaum G, Benvenisty AJ. Graft Acceptance: modification of immunogenicity of the donor or the donor organ with or without host immunosuppression. In Deltz A, Thiede A, Hammelmann H (eds.) *Small Bowel Transplantation*. Berlin, Springer-Verlag, pp. 135–52, 1987.
9. Snell GD. The Homograft Reaction. *Ann Rev Microbiol* 1957; **11,** 439–55.
10. Lafferty KJ, Prowse SJ. Theory and practice of immunoregulation by tissue treatment prior to transplantation. *World J Surg* 1984; **8,** 187–97.
11. Steinman RM, Gutchinov B, Witmer MD, Nussenzweig MC. Dendritic cells are the principal stimulators of the primary mixed leukocyte reaction in mice. *J Exp Med* 1983; **157,** 613–27.
12. Batchelor JR, Welsh KI, Maynard A, Burgos H. Failure of long surviving, passively enhanced kidney allografts to provoke T-dependent alloimmunity. I. Retransplant of (AS × AUG)F1 kidneys into secondary AS recipients. *J Exp Med* 1979; **150,** 455–64.
13. Lechler RI, Batchelor JR. Restoration of immunogenicity of passenger cell-depleted kidney allografts by the addition of donor strain dendritic cells. *J Exp Med* 1982; **155,** 31–41.
14. Lafferty KJ. Immunogenicity of foreign tissues. *Transplantation* 1980; **29,** 179–82.
15. Lafferty KJ, Cunningham AJ. A new analysis of allogeneic interactions. *Aust J Exp Bio Med Sci* 1975; **53,** 27–42.
16. Bretscher P, Cohn M. A theory of non-self discrimination. *Science* 1970; **169,** 1042–9.
17. Brandtzaeg P, Halstensen TS, Kett K, Krajci P, Kvale D, Rognum TO, Scott H, Sollid LM. Immunobiology and immunopathology of human gut mucosa: humoral immunity and intraepithelial lymphocytes. *Gastroenterology* 1989; **97,** 1562–84.
18. Wilders MM, Drexhage HA, Weltevreden EF, Mullink H, Duijvestijn A, Meuwissen SGM. Large mononuclear Ia-positive veiled cells in Peyer's patches. I. Isolation and characterization in rat, guinea pig and pig. *Immunology* 1983; **48,** 453–60.
19. Wilders MM, Sminia T, Plesch BEC, Drexhage HA, Weltevreden EF, Meuwissen SGM. Large mononuclear Ia-positive veiled cells in Peyer's patches. II. Localization in rat Peyer's patches. *Immunology* 1983; **48,** 461–7.
20. Wilders MM, Sminia T, Janse EM. Ontogeny of non-lymphoid and lymphoid cells in the rat gut with special reference to large mononuclear Ia-positive dendritic cells. *Immunology* 1983; **50,** 303–14.
21. Li X, Tucker J, Quan D, Duff J, Zhong R, Grant D. Alloantigen-presenting activity of cells from rat small intestine. *Transplant Proc* 1992; **24**(3), 1150.
22. Stone HB, Owings JC, Grey GO. Transplantation of living grafts of thyroid and parathyroid glands. *Annals Surg* 1934; **100,** 613–28.
23. Trowell OA. The sensitivity of lymphocytes to ionising radiation. *J Path Bact* 1952; **64,** 687–704.
24. Freeman JS, Chambulair EC, Reemtsma K, Steinmuller D. Prolongation of rat heart allograft by donor pretreatment with immunosuppressive agents. *Transplant Proc* 1971; **3,** 580–2.
25. Stuart FP, Garrick T, Holter A, Lynch A, Bastien E. Delayed rejection of renal allografts in the rat and dog by reduction of passenger leukocytes. *Surgery* 1971; **70,** 128–34.
26. Hume DM, Jackson BT, Zukoski CF, Lee HM, Kauffman HM, Egdahl RH. The homotransplantation of kidney and of fetal liver and spleen after total body irradiation. *Ann Surg* 1960; **152,** 354–73.
27. Steinmuller D, Warden G, Coleman M, Lofgreen J, Reemtsma K, Stuart F, Ganick T, Holter A, Lynch A. Prolonged survival of rat

the participation of immunologic components in transplantation, Schraut et al.[22] and Koltun et al.[23] found that rats receiving an intestinal graft with a systemic shunt had reduced body weight, moderate liver atrophy, increased ammonia levels, and abnormal amino acid profiles. Shaffer et al., however, could not see any difference in these measures during 6 weeks of pair-feeding.[24]

Using a heterotopic allotransplantation model from (LEW/BN)/F1 donors to LEW recipients, Schraut et al. and others studied the difference in immunologic responses between the two drainage methods.[25,26,27] Without immunosuppression, mean survival with a mesenteric-systemic shunt was 10.5 days, while it was significantly prolonged to 22.9 days in animals with portal intestinal drainage. Portal drainage appeared to suppress the early onset of acute rejection, but enhanced the development of chronic rejection. Although these findings supported the theory that transhepatic drainage of venous outflow mitigates the immune response to the intestinal graft, they were not confirmed in the experiment by Shaffer et al., using the same strain combination and surgical technique.[24] Neither group could find any immunologic benefit by transhepatic portal drainage when the intestinal transplantation was performed with a GVHD strain combination, LEW to (LEW/BN) F1, or with a bi-directional strain combination of BN to LEW.[24,27]

However, because animal survival is determined by the function of the recipient's own small bowel in the heterotopic intestinal transplantation model used by these investigators, we used an orthotopic transplantation technique with the BN to LEW strain combination.[28] When no immunosuppression was given, both group animals died of intestinal rejection with median survival time of 12.0 days in portal drainage animals and 10.5 days in systemic shunt animals (not significant). When a moderate dose of FK 506 was administered for two weeks postoperatively, all of the animals except for one in each group survived for more than 100 days. Although long-surviving animals from both groups showed similar histopathologic changes of chronic graft rejection, postoperative weight gain was superior when the venous drainage was transportal. These findings suggested that portal drainage of the intestinal graft offers better metabolic conditions, but provides little immunologic benefit.

Large animal experiments

Conflicting results also have been reported in large animal experiments. Using an autotransplantation model in dogs, Raju et al. studied the nutritional status, body weight, nitrogen balance, d-xylose and fat absorption, serum iron, and serum albumin for as long as one year.[29] Most of these measures except for body weight and nitrogen balance were abnormal with both portal and systemic venous drainage methods, but more severely so in the animals reconstructed with a mesenteric-systemic shunt. However, no such metabolic distinction was seen between the two drainage methods in the pig experiments of Kaneko et al.[30] In addition, the latter authors could not prove any prolongation of animal survival of portal drainage in allotransplantation experiments under treatment with cyclosporin.

Clinical experience

Historical cases

Detailed descriptions of operative procedures and postoperative courses of 11 patients receiving isolated intestinal grafts under azathioprine or cyclosporin have been reported by others in the literature (Table 10.2).[31–41] The arterial reconstruction in these cases was made by using three vessels: the infrarenal abdominal aorta, the iliac artery, and the superior mesenteric artery. The preferred outflow sites for intestinal venous drainage were the iliac vein and the inferior vena cava, but the left renal vein, the superior mesenteric vein and the portal vein were also used in three cases. In the selection of the recipient vein for these reconstructions, technical feasibility was the single most determining factor. For example, Alican anastomosed the graft vein to the left renal vein of the recipient since both the inferior vena cava and the iliac vein were completely thrombosed by his patient's underlying disease.

It was not practical to compare the performance of systemic versus portal drainage methods in these clinical cases because most of the grafts failed shortly after intestinal transplantation. However, it is noteworthy that two recipients whose graft venous flow (one from a segment of living donor intestine and the other a cadaver intestine) was drained into the systemic circulation, are currently alive for more than 3.5 and 4 years, respectively, with no evidence of metabolic abnormality.[39,41] One of the patients, a 15 month-

Table 10.2 Historical cases of isolated intestinal transplantation

Year	Investigator	Reference Number	Patient's Age	Indication	Donor	Graft	Reconstruction Artery	Reconstruction Vein
A. Azathioprine era								
1967	Lillehei	31	46	SMV thrombosis	Cadaveric	Whole	Iliac	Iliac
1968	Okumura	32	34	SMA thrombosis	Cadaveric	Partial	Iliac	Iliac
1969	Olivier	33	35	Gardner's syndrome	Cadaveric	Whole	SMA	SMV
1969	Allican	34	8	Volvulus	Living	Partial	Aorta	Left Renal
1970	Fortner	35	37	Gardner's syndrome	Living	Partial	Iliac	Iliac
B. Cyclosporine era								
1985	Cohen	36	26	Gardner's syndrome	Cadaveric	Whole	Aorta	IVC
1987	Goulet	37	9	Volvulus	Cadaveric	Partial	Aorta	IVC
1988	Hansmann	38	5	Volvulus	Living	Partial	Iliac	Iliac
1988	Deltz	39	42	SMV thrombosis	Living	Partial	Iliac	Iliac
1988	Grant	40	8	Neuromyopathy	Cadaveric	Whole	Aorta	Portal
1989	Goulet	41	0.4	Volvulus	Cadaveric	Whole	Aorta	IVC

old girl, who was underdeveloped at the time of transplantation, is now normal for both height and weight.[41] Thus, the problem of venous drainage in clinical intestinal transplantation may have less influence on metabolism and immunology than in animal experiments.

Our experience

We tried to drain the intestine physiologically through the host portal vein in our isolated intestinal recipients. The predicted technical difficulties were minimized by using a mesenteric piggy-back procedure.[42] With this approach, the portal vein is found in the subhepatic triad and dissected to obtain enough length for its side to accept the end of the superior mesenteric vein or the portal vein of the graft. This has been feasible even when the patients have had multiple laparotomies and adhesions. Of the 9 recipients in whom an isolated graft was transplanted, intestinal transplantation was successfully performed with this technique in 7. In the remaining two, the recipient superior mesenteric vein which was dissected out of the scar inferior to the transverse mesocolon was used to receive the graft superior mesenteric vein end-to-end. The inferior vena cava for mesenteric outflow was used on one occasion for retransplantation of a patient who had a gunshot wound at the hepatic hilum and who lost the first graft to chronic rejection. The venous drainage for the first graft had been via an end-to-end anastomosis to the recipient's superior mesenteric vein. There were no technical complications nor metabolic problems in any of these cases.

Liver in intestinal grafting

There are numerous experiments demonstrating that the concomitantly transplanted liver induces immunologic protection, or tolerance, to other organ allografts procured from the same donor. Because of severe graft rejection that develops in experimental and clinical intestinal transplantation, Grant et al. proposed that the liver should be transplanted with the intestinal graft to mitigate graft rejection, even if the recipient has normal liver function.[43] In contrast, patients who have intestinal failure and liver disease, as complication of TPN or inborn errors, require combined intestine and liver transplant. If the intestinal failure is from the thrombotic problems that involve both the celiac axis and the superior mesenteric artery or if the indication is a centrally located tumour, abdominal multivisceral transplantation may be chosen as the method of surgical treatment.

Basic considerations

Hepatic tolerogenicity

Evidence of hepatic tolerogenicity for other tissues and organs from the same donor was first noted in our original canine multivisceral experiments.[44] The concept was fully developed by Calne in 1969 who showed indefinite prolongation of kidney and skin graft survival in pigs receiving concomitant liver transplantation.[45] This finding was confirmed later by Kamada and others, using rat liver transplantation with various strain combinations.[46] The mechanism of hepatic tolerogenicity is still unclear, but many explanations have been proposed, such as clonal deletion of cytotoxic T cells, production of antibody to class II MHC, liver enzymes inactivating antigen, antigen alteration by Kuppfer cells, inhibition of immune stimulation, and production of soluble donor class I antigen. However, the recent demonstration that migratory tissue leukocytes from the liver create a state of microchimerism in the recipient has provided an alternative and more likely explanation.[47,48,49]

Microchimerism

We now believe that the development of two-way cell traffic, between the graft and the recipient, leading to long-lasting systemic microchimerism is the reason for hepatic tolerance as well as tolerance induced by other organs including the intestine. During histoimmunologic studies of rats receiving multivisceral transplantation, Murase et al. found that the cells in the lymphoid and non-lymphoid tissues of the grafts were replaced by recipient-derived cells as early as 12 days after transplant,[50] a finding also seen by Arnaud-Battandier in pigs.[51] Not only did recipient spindle-shaped dendritic cells, positive for anti-recipient-Ia monoclonal antibody, repopulate into the graft, but donor dendritic cells migrated from the graft and resided in tissues of the recipient.[52] After intestinal transplantation, donor-derived cells in the spleen, mesenteric lymph nodes and peripheral blood in the recipient accounted approximately for 10–15 per cent of cells at 1 week, 5–10 per cent at 3 weeks and 5 per cent at 4 to 6 weeks.[52] Similarly, Iwaki et al. described two-way cell traffic phenomenon in the patients receiving intestinal transplantation.[53] Ten to 15 per cent of peripheral blood cells in the human recipients were of donor phenotype for several weeks after transplantation, and lymphoid tissues of the intestinal graft were completely repopulated by recipient-derived cells within 45–90 days after transplantation. Although Grant attributed the presence of donor cells in recipient circulation to transient GVHD,[43] no GVHD was seen in Iwaki's cases and we now realize that this occurs in all cases.

The two-way cell traffic phenomenon or microchimerism is not unique to intestinal transplantation, but is also seen after transplantation of other organs in both experimental and clinical settings; donor-derived dendritic cells were demonstrated in the peripheral blood and tissues of patients who underwent hepatic or renal transplantation 10 to 29 years previously. Thus, development of systemic chimerism seems to be an obligatory step for successful transplantation and for graft acceptance or tolerance in all whole organs. These findings suggest that the liver exhibits more pronounced tolerogenicity because it contains abundant lymphoreticular cells and has a greater capacity to induce systemic microchimerism than other organs. Donor-specific soluble class I antigens that are detectable in systemic circulation after liver transplantation have been attributed to hepatocytes,[54] but these antigens undoubtedly are secreted in large part by these peripheralized donor-derived cells of macrophage/monocyte lineage.

Experimental findings with intestinal transplantation

Rat experiments

Protection by the liver of intestinal graft rejection has been studied by Grant's group in Canada and Goulet's group in France.[55,56,57] Grant et al. demonstrated that when the LEW intestine was transplanted into DA rats without immunosuppression, all of the rats developed histologic acute rejection at 7 days, and had full-thickness necrosis of the intestinal wall at 14 days at sacrifice. However, these changes were not observed when they transplanted the intestine and liver simultaneously. Combined graft recipients had suppressed function of both T and B cells. Goulet and his associates tried to induce tolerance of the intestine by transplanting the intestine 14 days after liver transplantation from DA rats to PVD rats.[57] By this method, five of the six combined graft animals lived for more than 150 days without any immunosuppression, whereas all of the isolated intestine recipients died of rejection with median animal survival of 7.6 days.

However, the induction of immunologic protection by the liver appears to be limited to particular strain combinations and to the timing of intestinal grafting after liver transplantation. When the combined grafts from DA rats were transplanted simultaneously,[56] not separately, into PVG recipients (a low responder), the intestine did not become tolerant; rather, the PVG recipients died within 9 days after transplant from lethal GVHD. Neither the liver nor intestine of the combined graft animals showed rejection. Animals receiving an isolated graft of this combination died by rejection with mean survival of 18.6 days. When a BN to LEW combination (a moderate responder) was used, animals that received a combined graft died either of GVHD or liver rejection with mean survival of 12.6 days. Isolated intestinal graft recipients with this combination died of rejection with a mean survival time of 12.8 days. Finally, when an ACI to LEW combination (a high responder) was used, 3 out of the 5 combined graft animals died within 13 days from severe hepatic rejection but with normal intestine. Isolated graft rats in this combination died of rejection with mean survival of 12 days.

Instead of combined intestine and liver grafts, we studied immunologic protection by the liver using a multivisceral transplantation model in BN to LEW strain combination.[50,58] The results of multivisceral transplantation were compared with those with isolated intestine or liver transplantation alone. Without immunosuppression, isolated liver recipients survived indefinitely, whereas animals receiving multiple organs or an isolated intestine lived only for 10 to 13 days. Both groups of animals had severe and similar intestinal rejection by histopathologic study. Thus, immunologic protection by the liver to the companion intestine was not demonstrated in this model. When a 14-day course treatment with low-dose FK 506 was given, most of the animals were able to survive for more than a 100 days in all three transplant groups.[50] However, intestinal rejection detected by histologic analysis of sacrificed animals was worse in animals with an isolated intestine than in animals with a composite of multivisceral grafts. Body weight gain was suppressed in isolated graft animals compared with the multivisceral group. These findings indicate that the liver in the multivisceral graft provides an immunologic advantage to the companion intestine under low-dose FK 506 treatment. However, when immunosuppression was augmented to a high-dose 14-day course therapy, the difference between the multivisceral group and the isolated intestine group decreased. When both groups of animals were treated by high-dose FK 506 for 14 days and with weekly supplementation, there was no difference in body weight gain or histologic severity of intestinal rejection. Hepatic tolerogenicity that is barely seen with low-dose immunosuppression became insignificant when high-dose FK 506 was administered.

Large animal experiments

The multivisceral transplant operation was described in dogs more than 30 years ago.[44] Of the 38 animals submitted to this operation in 1959 without immunosuppression, only 5 lived for 5.5 to 9 days. Histologic studies revealed attenuation of liver graft rejection in these animals compared with animals that underwent liver transplantation alone, suggesting mitigation of the rejection process. There also was little evidence of rejection in the bowel and other organs of the multivisceral graft, prompting the conclusion that here also rejection was attenuated. On the other hand, strong histopathologic evidence of GVH reaction was found in the bone marrow, lungs, and other organs of the animals receiving multivisceral organs than in animals receiving isolated liver grafts.

Clinical experience

Historical cases

In November 1987, a child in Pittsburgh who received a multivisceral graft became the first recipient of an intestine that provided nutritional function. The patient died after 6 months of a B cell lymphoma, but during life there was little or no evidence of rejection – either of the liver or of the other viscera.[59] Immunosuppression was with cyclosporin, low doses of prednisone, and OKT3.

More decisive clinical evidence of amelioration of intestinal rejection by a hepatic graft was subsequently described by Grant et al. in a 41 year-old woman, who lost her small intestine by superior mesenteric artery thrombosis from antithrombin-III deficiency.[43] She received a combined liver and small bowel allograft under immunosuppression with cyclosporin, steroids and azathioprine. The donor was treated by OKT3 before procurement. After surgery, she developed mild GVHD on the eleventh postoperative day, which subsided spontaneously. During the ninth postoperative week, she developed mild intestinal rejection which was easily treated by steroid tapering and OKT3. There was no other episode of rejection in either of the grafts thereafter. The patient has been doing well for the past 4 years, nutritionally supported by an unlimited oral diet. The benign postoperative course in this historically important case was in clear contrast to this group's previous experiences with clinical intestinal transplantation, suggesting that the co-existing liver graft ameliorated intestinal rejection. However, a patient who received a combined graft in Wisconsin died after 52 days by rejection,[60] and a second patient treated by us with multivisceral transplantation under cyclosporin suffered the same fate as well as a disseminated lymphoma.[61]

Our experience

We only perform a combined intestine and liver transplant on patients who have end-stage organ failure in both the intestine and liver. Of the 17 recipients receiving combined grafts at our centre under FK 506-based immunosuppression, all had cholestatic liver disease related to long-term hyperalimentation, with a median preoperative serum bilirubin level of 18.5 mg/dl, ranging from 2.3 mg/dl to 50.5 mg/dl. Most of these patients had evident portal hypertension and hypersplenism. Nine patients who had intestinal failure with normal liver function were transplanted with the intestine alone. Twelve out of the 17 combined graft recipients and all of the isolated graft recipients were operated on between May 1990 and June 1992. The survival, postoperative course, and the incidence and severity of graft rejection with a minimum follow-up for three months were computed and compared to determine the performance of respective surgical procedures (Table 10.3).[62,63]

Nine of the 12 combined graft recipients are currently alive. There were 3 deaths: 2 from septic complications related to technical problems and 1 from postoperative lymphoproliferative disease. Patient and graft survival was 75 per cent (9/12). Of the 9 isolated graft recipients, one patient died from sepsis 71 days after retransplantation and removal of the primary graft which had been destroyed by chronic rejection after 23 months. Another patient required graft removal and re-turned to hyperalimentation after discontinuation of immunosuppression because of viral encephalitis. Patient and graft survival was 88.9 per cent (8/9) and 70 per cent (7/10), respectively.

Table 10.3 Comparison of intestinal graft performance

	Isolated small bowel	**Combined small bowel and liver**
Number		
Patient	9	12
Graft	10	12
Survival*		
Patient	8 (90%)	9 (75%)
Graft	7 (70%)	9 (75%)
ICU Stay, days	6 (4–14)	3 (3–300)
Hospital Stay, days	79 (33–159)	82 (23–320)
Readmission, times	1 (1–7)	2.5 (0–9)
Stop TPN, days	30 (19–113)	83.5 (44–330)
Rejection Episodes		
Intestine	10 (90%)	10 (83%)
Current Status		
TPN, Free	7	8
TPN, Partial	1	1
Hospital	2	0
Home	6	8

*Follow-up till 30 September 1992

The postoperative courses, including Intensive Care Unit (ICU) stay, hospital stay, start of enteral feeding, and discontinuation of TPN, were more favourable for isolated graft recipients than those with the combined grafts. Methods of monitoring and treating graft rejection have been described elsewhere.[2–5,64] Of the 22 grafts, 19 experienced intestinal rejection. This occurred at a 90 per cent incidence (9/10) in the isolated grafts and at an incidence of 83 per cent (10/12) when the intestine was part of a combination graft (differences not significant). Of the 12 combined grafts, acute rejection was more frequent with the intestine (83 per cent, 10/12) than in the liver (42 per cent, 5/12). The incidence of liver rejection in the combined graft was not different from that seen after liver transplantation alone. Synchronous graft rejection in the combined grafts (diagnosed by biopsy samples) of the small intestine and liver was seen on 8 occasions: this accounted for 17 per cent of 48 episodes of intestinal rejection versus 31 per cent of 26 episodes of hepatic rejection. In contrast, 83 per cent (40/48) and 69 per cent (18/26) of the total episodes of acute rejection developed independently in intestine and in liver, respectively.

Conclusions

Our experience has shown that clinical transplantation of the intestine alone or with other abdominal viscera is feasible under the improved immunosuppression that has been made possible with FK 506. How much these procedures can improve the quality of life for patients who are destined to remain on TPN for life, or save patients from lethal TPN-related complications, will have to be determined by more cases and longer follow-up periods. Venous outflow from isolated intestinal grafts can be drained into the portal system and then through the native liver using a mesenteric piggy-back method. If the mesenteric piggy-back method is not possible, a mesenteric-systemic shunt can be used, probably without serious metabolic consequences. Although hepatic tolerogenicity is a well-established concept, simultaneous liver transplantation is not necessary for successful intestinal transplantation in humans and it adds to the risk and magnitude of the treatment if the patient does not have hepatic failure. Thus, isolated intestinal transplantation should be chosen for patients who are destined to be on TPN for life, but who still have normal liver function. Combined intestine and liver transplantation is reserved for those patients who need an intestine and have liver failure as a complication of TPN or inborn hepatic disorders. Multivisceral transplantation is reserved for special indications.

References

1. Grant D. Intestinal transplantation: current status. *Transplant Proc* 1989; **21,** 2869–71.
2. Starzl TE, Todo S, Tzakis A, Alessiani M, Casavilla A, Abu-Elmagd K, Fung JJ. The many faces of multivisceral transplantation. *Surg Gynecol Obstet* 1991; **172,** 335–44.
3. Tzakis AG, Todo S, Reyes J, Starzl TE. Liver and small bowel transplantation for short gut syndrome in a child. *Transplant Sci* 1991; **1,** 17–33.
4. Todo S, Tzakis AG, Abu-Elmagd K, Reyes J, Fung JJ, Nakamura K, Yagihashi A, Jain A, Murase N, Iwaki Y, Demetris AJ, Van Thiel DH, Starzl TE. Cadaveric small bowel and small bowel–liver transplantation in humans. *Transplantation* 1992; **53,** 369–76.
5. Todo S, Tzakis AG, Abu-Elmagd K, Reyes J, Nakamura K, Casavilla A, Selby R, Nour BM, Wright H, Fung JJ, Demetris AJ, Van Thiel DH, Starzl TE. Intestinal transplantation in composite visceral grafts or alone. *Ann Surg* 1992; **216,** 223–34.
6. Casavilla A, Selby R, Abu-Elmagd K, Tzakis A, Todo S, Reyes J, Fung J, Starzl TE. Logistics and technique for combined hepatic-intestinal retrieval. *Ann Surg* 1992; **216,** 85–9.
7. Starzl TE, Porter KA, Francavilla A. The eck fistula in animals and humans. *Curr Prob Surg* 1983; **20,** 692–745.
8. Lindstedt S. The turnover of cholic acid in man. *Acta Physiol Scand* 1957; **40,** 1–9.
9. Stange EF, Dietchy JM. Cholesterol absorption and metabolism. In Danielsson H, Sjövall J (ed.) *Steroids and Bile Acids*. Amsterdam: Elsevier, pp. 121–5, 1985.
10. Summerskill WHJ, Wolpert E. Ammonia metabolism in the gut. *Am J Clin Nutr* 1970; **23,** 633–9.
11. Marchioro TL, Porter KA, Brown BI, et al. The effect of partial portacaval transposition on the canine liver. *Surgery* 1967; **61,** 723–32.
12. Starzl TE, Porter KA, Watanabe K, et al. The effects of insulin, glucagon and insulin/glucagon infusions upon liver morphology and cell division after complete portacaval shunt in dogs. *Lancet* 1976; **1,** 821–5.
13. Francavilla A, Starzl TE, Porter K, Scotti-Foglieni C, Michalopoulos GK, Carrieri G, Trejo J, Azzarone A, Barone M, Zeng Q. Screening for candidate hepatic growth factors by selective portal infusion after canine eck fistula. *Hepatology* 1991; **14,** 665–70.
14. Mandel MA, Monaco AP, Russel PS. Destruction of splenic transplantation antigens by a factor present in the liver. *J Immunol* 1965; **95,** 673–82.
15. Holman JM Jr, Todd R. Enhanced survival of heterotopic rat heart allografts with portal venous drainage. *Transplantation* 1990; **49,** 229–30.
16. Mazzoni G, DiMartino C, Demofonti A, et al. A comparison of portal and systemic venous drainage in porcine renal allografts. *Br J Surg* 1972; **59,** 541–4.
17. Pfefferman R, Sakai A, Kountz SL. The liver as a privileged site for parathyroid alloimplantation in the rat. *Surgery* 1976; **79,** 182–7.
18. Eloy R, Kedinger M, Garaud K, et al. Isogenic and allogenic transplantation of isolated langerhans islets into the liver. *Lang Arch Chir* 1975; **109** (suppl), 109–14.
19. Sakai A. Role of the liver in kidney allograft rejection in the rat. *Transplantation* 1970; **9,** 333–4.
20. Boeckx W, Sobis H, Laquet A, et al. Prolongation of allogenic heart graft survival in the rat after im-

plantation on portal vein. *Transplantation* 1975; **19,** 145–9.
21. Mazzoni G, Benichou J, Porter KA, et al. Renal homotransplantation with venous outflow or infusion of antigen into the portal vein of dogs or pigs. *Transplantation* 1977; **24,** 268–73.
22. Schraut WH, Abraham VS, Loe KKW. Portal versus caval venous drainage of small bowel allografts: Technical and metabolic consequences. *Surgery* 1986; **99,** 193–8.
23. Koltun WA, Madara JL, Smith RJ, Kirkman RL. Metabolic aspects of small bowel transplantation in inbred rats. *J Surg Res* 1987; **42,** 341–7.
24. Shaffer D, Diflo T, Love W, Clowes GHA, Maki T, Monaco AP. Immunologic and metabolic effects of caval versus portal venous drainage in small-bowel transplantation. *Surgery* 1988; **104,** 518–24.
25. Schraut WH, Rosemurgy AS, Riddle RM. Prolongation of intestinal allograft survival without immunosuppressive drug therapy: Transplantation of small bowel allografts. *J Surg Res* 1983; **34,** 597–607.
26. Rosemurgy AS, Schraut WH. Small bowel allografts: Sequence of histologic changes in acute and chronic rejection. *Am J Surg* 1986; **151,** 470–5.
27. Schraut WH, Abraham VS, Lee KKW. Portal versus systemic venous drainage for small-bowel allografts. *Surgery* 1985; **98**, 579–85.
28. Murase N, Demetris AJ, Furuya T, Todo S, Fung JJ, Starzl TE. Comparison of the small intestine after multivisceral transplantation and the small intestine transplanted with portal versus caval drainage. *Transplant Proc* 1992; **24,** 1143–4.
29. Raju S, Fujiwara H, Grogan JB, Achord JL. Long-term nutritional function of orthotopic small bowel autotransplants. *J Surg Res* 1989; **46,** 142–6.
30. Kaneko H, Fischman MA, Buckley TM, Schweizer RT. A comparison of portal versus systemic venous drainage in the pig small-bowel allograft recipient. *Surgery* 1991; **109,** 663–70.
31. Lillehei RC, Idezuki Y, Feemster JA, Dietzman RH, Kelly WD, Merkel FK, Goetz FC, Lyons GW, Manax WG. Transplantation of stomach, intestine and pancreas: Experimental and clinical observations. *Surgery* 1967; **62,** 721–41.
32. Okumura M, Fujimura I, Ferrari AA, Nakiri K, Lemos PCP, de Andrea EA, Bahdur R, Marek SR, Neto MJY, Posso BJM, Fonseca JF, Iriya K, Antonascio F, de Faria JF, Magaldi JDB, de Paula W, Raia AA. Transplante de Intestino Delgado: apresentaçao de um caso. *Rev Hosp Clin Fac Med S Paulo* 1969; **2D,** 39–54.
33. Olivier Cl, Rettori R, Olivier CH, Baur O, Roux J. Homotransplantation orthotopique de l'intestin grêle et des côlons droit en transverse chez l'homme. *J Chir (Paris)* 1969; **98,** 323–30.
34. Alican F, Hardy JD, Cayirli M, Varner JE, Moynihan PC, Turner MD, Anas P. Intestinal Transplantation: Laboratory Experience and Report of a Clinical Case. *Am J Surg* 1971; **121,** 105–7.
35. Fortner JG, Sichuk G, Litwin SD, Beattie EJ Jr. Immunological responses to an intestinal allograft with HL-A-identical donor-recipient. *Transplantation* 1972; **14,** 531–5.
36. Cohen Z, Silverman RE, Wassef R, et al. Small intestinal transplantation using cyclosporine: report of a case. *Transplantation* 1986; **42,** 613.
37. Goulet OJ, Révillon Y, Cerf-Bensussan N, Nezelof C, Fischer A, Buisson C, Hubert P, Lokiec F, Martelli H, Niaudet P, Jan D, Pellerin D, Ricour C. Small intestinal transplantation in a child using cyclosporine. *Transplant Proc* 1988; **20,** 288–96.
38. Hansmann ML, Deltz E, Gundlach M, Schroeder P, Radzun HJ. Small bowel transplantation in a child. *Am J Clin Pathol* 1989; **92**, 686–92.
39. Deltz E, Schroeder P, Gebhardt H, Gundlach M, Timmermann W, Engemann R, Leimenstoll G, Hansmann ML, Westphal E, Hamelmann H. Successful clinical small bowel transplantation: report of a case. *Clin Transplant* 1989; **3,** 89–91.
40. Grant D, Sommerauer J, Mimeault R, Garcia B, Ghent C, Zhong R, Stiller C, Duff J. Treatment with continuous high-dose intravenous cyclosporine following clinical intestinal transplantation. *Transplantation* 1989; **48,** 151–2.
41. Goulet O, Revillon Y, Brousse N, Jan D, Canion D, Rambaud C, Cerf-Bensussan N, Buisson C, Hubert P, De Potter S, Mougenot JF, Fischer A, Ricour C. Successful small bowel transplantation in an infant. *Transplantation* 1992; **53,** 940–3.
42. Tzakis AG, Todo S, Reyes J, Nour B, Fung JJ, Starzl TE. Piggyback orthotopic intestinal transplantation. *Surg Gynecol Obstet* 1993; **176**(3), 297–8.
43. Grant D, Wall W, Mimeault R, Zhong R, Ghent C, Garcia B, Stiller C, Duff J. Successful small-bowel/liver transplantation. *Lancet* 1990; **335,** 181–4.
44. Starzl TE, Kaupp HA Jr, Brock DR, Butz GW Jr, Linman JW. Homotransplantation of multiple visceral organs. *Am J Surg* 1962; **103,** 219–9.
45. Calne RY, Sells RA, Pena, et al. Induction of immunological tolerance by porcine liver allografts. *Nature* 1969; **223,** 472–6.
46. Kamada N, Davies HS, Wight D, Culank L, Roser B. Liver transplantation in the rat: Biochemical and histological evidence of complete tolerance induction in non-rejector strains. *Transplantation* 1983; **35,** 304–11.
47. Starzl TE, Demetris AJ, Murase N, Ildstad S, Ricordi C, Trucco M. Cell migration, chimerism and graft acceptance. *Lancet* 1992; **339,** 1579–82.
48. Starzl TE, Demetris AJ, Trucco M, Ramos H,

Zeevi A, Rudert WA, Kocoua M, Ricordi C, Ildstad S, Murase N. Systemic chimerism in human female recipients of male livers. *Lancet* 1992; **340,** 876–7.

49. Starzl TE, Demetris AJ, Trucco M, Ricordi S, Ildstad S, Terasaki P, Murase N, Kendall RS, Kocoua M, Rudert WA, Zeevi A, Van Thiel D. Chimerism after liver transplantation for type IV glycogen storage disease and Type I Gaucher's disease. *N Engl J Med* 1993; **328,** 745–9.
50. Murase N, Demetris AJ, Matsuzaki T, Yagihasi A, Todo S, Fung J, Starzl TE. Long survival in rats after multivisceral versus isolated small bowel allotransplantation under FK 506. *Surgery* 1991; **110,** 87–98.
51. Arnaud-Baltandier F, Salmon H, Vaiman H, et al. Small intestinal allotransplantation swine with cyclosporine treatment: studies of the lymphoid population. *Transplant Proc* 1985; **17,** 1440–2.
52. Murase N, Demetris AJ, Woo J, Tanabe M, Furuya T, Todo S, Starzl TE. Graft versus host disease (GVHD) after BN to LEW compared to LEW to BN intestinal transplantation under FK 506. *Transplantation* 1993; **55,** 1–7.
53. Iwaki Y, Starzl TE, Yagihashi A, Taniwaki S, Abu-Elmagd K, Tzakis A, Fung J, Todo S. Replacement of donor lymphoid tissue in human small bowel transplants under FK 506 immunosuppression. *Lancet* 1991; **337,** 818–19.
54. Davies HFFS, Pollard SG, Calne RY. Soluble HLA antigens in the circulation of liver graft recipients. *Transplantation* 1989; **47,** 524–7.
55. Zhong R, Gang H, Sakai Y, Li XC, Garcia B, Wall W, Duff J, Stiller C, Grant D. Combined small bowel and liver transplantation in the rat: Possible role of the liver in preventing intestinal allograft rejection. *Transplantation* 1991; **52,** 550–76.
56. Zhong R, He G, Sakai Y, Zhang Z, Quan D, Garcia B, Duff J, Grant D. The effect of donor –recipient strain combinations in combined liver/intestine transplantation in the rat. *Transplant Proc* 1992; **24,** 1208–9.
57. Sarnacki S, Révillon Y, Cerf-Bensussan N, Calise D, Goulet O, Brousse N. Long-term small-bowel graft survival induced by a spontaneously tolerated liver allograft in inbred rat strains. *Transplantation* 1992; **54,** 383–5.
58. Murase N, Demetris AJ, Kim DG, Todo S, Fung JJ, Starzl TE. Rejection of the multivisceral allografts in rats: A sequential analysis with comparison to isolated orthotopic small bowel and liver grafts. *Surgery* 1990; **108,** 880–9.
59. Starzl TE, Rowe M, Todo S, Jaffe R, Tzakis A, Hoffman A, Esquivel C, Porter K, Venkataramanan R, Makowka L, Duquesnoy R. Transplantation of multiple abdominal viscera. *J Am Med Assn* 1989; **26,** 1449–57.
60. D'Alessandro AM, Kalayoglu M, Sollinger HW, Pirsch JD, Belzer FO. Liver-intestinal transplantation: Report of a case. *Transplant Proc* 1992; **24,** 1228–9.
61. Jaffe R, Trager JDK, Zeevi A, Sonmez-Alpan E, Duquesnoy R, Todo S, Rowe M, Starzl TE. Multivisceral intestinal transplantation: Surgical pathology. *Pediatr Pathol* 1989; **9,** 633–54.
62. Abu-Elmagd K, Tzakis A, Todo S, Reyes J, Fung J, Nakamura K, Wright H, Furukawa H, Demetris J, Van Thiel DH, Starzl TE. Monitoring and treatment of intestinal allograft rejection in humans. *Transplant Proc* 1993; **25,** 1202–3.
63. Reyes J, Tzakis AG, Todo S, Nour B, Casavilla A, Abu-Elmagd K, Fung JJ, Starzl TE. Nutritional management of intestinal transplant recipients. *Transplant Proc* 1993; **25,** 1202–3.
64. Abu-Elmagd K, Fung JJ, Reyes J, Casavilla A, Van Thiel DH, Iwaki Y, Warty V, Nikolaidis N, Block J, Nakamura K, Goldbach B, Demetris J, Tzakis A, Todo S, Starzl TE. Management of intestinal transplantation in humans. *Transplant Proc* 1992; **24,** 1243–4.

11

Pathology of human intestinal transplantation

Olivier Goulet, Nicole Brousse, Yann Revillon and Claude Ricour

Introduction

Early diagnosis of rejection and effective treatment are essential, otherwise graft survival is compromised. In this chapter we review the main pathological aspects of isolated small bowel transplantation in paediatric patients receiving cyclosporin as the major component of their immunosuppressive regimen. In clinical small bowel transplantation, although graft-versus-host disease (GVHD) is a potential problem, acute rejection has been the predominant response.

Background

Isolated clinical small bowel transplantation was first reported by Lillehei et al. in 1967.[1] Before cyclosporin (CyA) became available, the 8 attempts at clinical small bowel transplantation were unsuccessful because of technical problems, sepsis, graft rejection or GVHD.[1–6] The longest survivor died after 76 days without adequate graft function.

Improved small intestinal allograft survival in experimental animals receiving CyA has been reported from several laboratories and has allowed new attempts in humans.[7–12] Cohen et al. in 1986 reported small bowel transplantation in an adult patient using a combination of CyA and corticosteroids;[13] the patient died 12 days after transplantation from haemodynamic disorders and encephalopathy. During the last 7 years, most attempts of isolated small bowel transplantation have failed because of severe, uncontrolled rejection despite powerful immunosuppressive drugs, including CyA, antilymphoglobulins, and OKT3 monoclonal antibody. In other patients, graft failure was related to complications of immunosuppression, which were often lethal. Thus, only 2 recipients (one had a living-related donor) of about 16 paediatric or adult patients with isolated small bowel grafts and CyA treatment have a functional graft more than 3.5 years after transplantation.[14,15] These poor results contrast with the recent success of liver/small bowel transplantation using CyA or FK 506 and isolated small bowel transplantation using FK 506.[16–19]

The Paris series

In our series of nine HLA-mismatched, isolated cadaveric small bowel transplants, the first transplant was marked by early necrosis of the graft, which was removed within 8 hours. Severe haemodynamic disorders, occurring just after unclamping, led to another patient's death 20 hours later. Our other patients recovered normal intestinal transit while graft stomal inspection became progressively normal.

When the proximal end of the graft is anastomosed to the native bowel, transit recovery is usually achieved within 24–48 hours postoperatively, with the appearance of biliary ileal output. In the absence of graft rejection, ileostomal drainage stabilizes around 100–300 ml every 24 hours. Nevertheless, in paediatric recipients with neonatal short bowel syndrome, a small abdominal cavity and larger graft volume led to complications. Indeed, one infant's postoperative course was marked by the absence of early ileostomal output and was accompanied by severe abdominal pressure and abundant gastric drainage. Ileal output appeared and increased at 6 days post-transplant. As abdominal pressure may compromise graft vascularization, graft length and volume should be tailored to recipient size.

The effect of preservation on graft histology

Retrieval and storage of the small bowel graft includes vascular flushing using 4°C Collins solution or University of Wisconsin solution (UW), sometimes with luminal washing.[17–20] Graft specimens, taken before and after revascularization, may be assessed by conventional histological and immunohistochemical techniques. Biopsies of grafts with less than 7 hours of cold ischaemia, using Collins or UW, showed no significant damage from graft preservation.[20,21] An increased HLA-DR expression on crypt enterocytes, observed before unclamping is probably related to ischaemia as this phenomenon was also reported in rat kidney grafts.[22] Although its role in the occurrence of graft rejection is unclear, increased epithelial DR expression should be considered when diagnosing graft rejection based on mucosal changes of further biopsies.[23] Grafts stored more than 7.5 hours revealed focal epithelial denudation of the villi and haemorrhage/congestion in the lamina propria, which healed within 10 days post-transplant.[21]

Acute graft rejection

Clinical signs

Early acute rejection occurs within the first 15 days following transplantation. In our experience, clinical symptoms appeared well after the first signs of histological damage. Thus, mild changes in either stomal output or the appearance of the ileostomy should be taken seriously. An increase in volume and sodium concentration (> 130 mEq/l) are related to mucosal lesions with decreased absorption of water and electrolytes. Close monitoring of stomal output, with assessment every 6 hours, is essential. Clinical symptoms, such as cyanotic changes of the stoma, haemorrhagic losses, abdominal pain with ileus and/or fever, follow within a few days and indicate severe graft rejection with major mucosal necrosis. Haemodynamic disorders, acidosis, or even septic shock from bacterial translocation can be observed at this stage.[17,19] By using total digestive decontamination of the graft during the early postoperative course, we have not encountered such septic complications.[20]

Diagnosis of graft rejection

Numerous techniques to detect graft rejection have been proposed in animal models[24–31] as well as in humans.[32–4] Methods include absorption tests, intestinal permeability and bacterial translocation, hyaluronan quantification, electrophysiological monitoring, measurements of monocyte procoagulant activity, serum N-acetyl hexoaminidase, and full-thickness biopsy with histochemical staining for enzymatic activity. Decreased activity of brush-border alkaline phosphatase or sucrase-isomaltase was thought to be an early sign of graft rejection;[35] in our experience, the first histological lesions were limited to the crypts and changes in alkaline phosphatase activity occurred later.

Early rejection has a patchy distribution in both humans and animals.[36] The necessity of initiating appropriate immunosuppressive therapy or removing the graft to salvage the recipient requires rapid and specific assessment of the rejection process. In the absence of specific early clinical or biological signs of graft rejection, histological and immunohistochemical studies of repeated graft biopsies are essential to detect graft rejection and guide immunosuppressive therapy. Stomal or upper gastrointestinal endoscopy is helpful for taking biopsy specimens. Visualization of the lumen is also useful for showing macroscopic changes of mucosal injury and loss of motility. In the adult experience reported by the transplant programme at Pittsburgh, USA,[37] graft rejection, using early endoscopic biopsies, was characterized by lack of peristalsis, oedema of the mucosa followed by pale mucosa, mucosal ulceration, and liquid enteric contents. Finally, they observed loss of mucosal pattern, mucosal sloughing and bleeding. Endoscopy is certainly a valuable tool in the management of adult intestinal recipients. However, histological examination and immunohistochemical tests are essential to detect changes preceding clinical and endoscopic signs of rejection. In our experience with paediatric patients, biopsy specimens were taken using H. Noblett Forceps or by upper gastrointestinal endoscopy (Olympus® GIF-XP-10). Biopsy specimens were processed for routine histology using paraffin sections, or frozen for immunohistochemistry. An indirect immunoperoxidase technique was applied to define the phenotype of the immune cells infiltrating the graft.[38] The monoclonal antibodies (MAb) used were anti-CD3 (Leu 4), anti-CD4 (Leu 3a), anti-CD8 (Leu 2a), anti-CD25 (IL2R), anti-HLA-DR from Becton Dickinson®, anti-CD68 (Ki-M7) (activated macrophages) from Behring®, and Ki-67 (proliferating cells) from Dakopatts®.

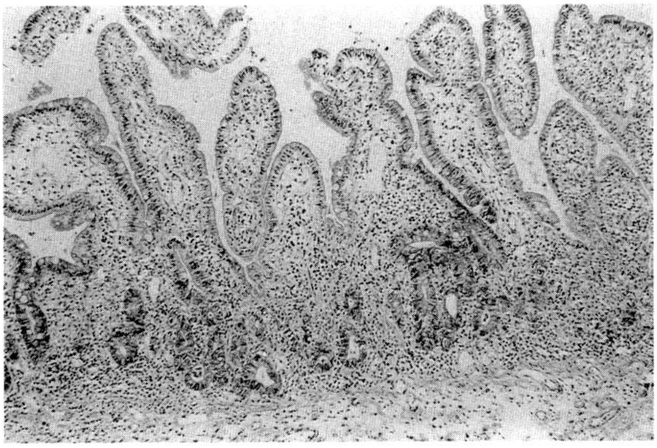

Fig. 11.1a Early histological changes suggest acute graft rejection appearing at day 12: villus oedema, increased number of mononuclear cells in the lamina propria around the crypts, and some necrotic glands.

Conventional histology

Using haematoxylin and eosin staining, mucosal changes initially included villous oedema and mononuclear cell infiltration into the lamina propria (Fig. 11.1a). Later, villous atrophy occurs with crypt epithelium necrosis and abrasion associated with an increased mixed cellular lamina propia (LP) infiltrate. This infiltrate consists primarily of lymphocytes with focal venulitis and cryptitis (Fig. 11.1b). Reparative epithelial changes such as irregularly-shaped lumens, mucus or Paneth cell depletion, and nuclear stratification were also described.[21] Finally, in the absence of graft rejection treatment, architectural distortions appear with villous blunting progressing to total disappearance of the epithelial surface and severe LP infiltration with lymphocytes and macrophages (Fig. 11.1C). Focal ulceration with resultant neutrophil plugging of capillaries and pseudomembrane formation with bacterial colonies were also reported.[21] At that point, patients are at risk of both:

1. *protein-losing enteropathy*, requiring electrolytes, haemoglobin, and albumin compensation, and
2. *bacterial translocation*, which may be prevented by digestive decontamination.

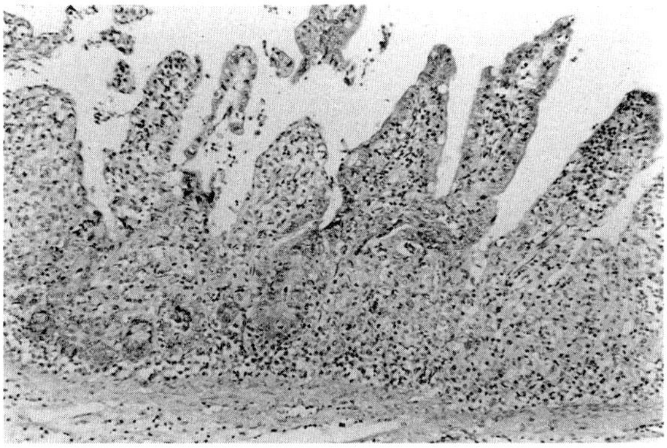

Fig. 11.1b Acute rejection with intense infiltration of the lamina propria and disappearance or necrosis of the epithelial crypts (twelfth day post-transplant). Persistence of the villi with epithelial necrosis.

Immunohistochemistry

In our experience, early and rapid diagnosis of graft rejection (within 2 hours) can be achieved by repeatedly performing immunohistochemical

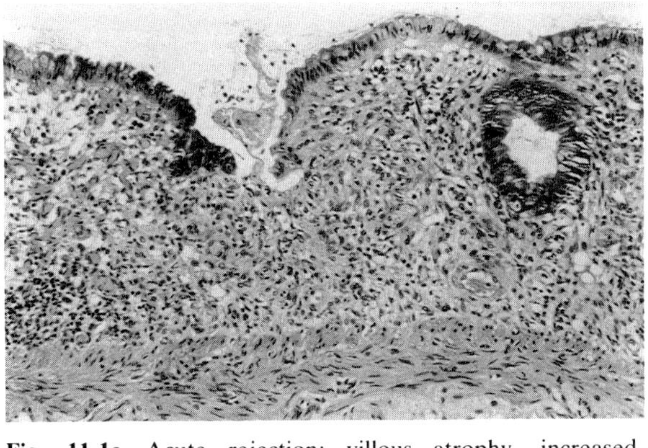

Fig. 11.1c Acute rejection: villous atrophy, increased number of mononuclear cells in the lamina propria and crypt necrosis or disappearance.

tests on biopsies obtained through the graft stoma and/or by upper gastrointestinal endoscopy.[23] In the absence of any morphological changes, immunohistochemical patterns include (i) appearance of pericryptic CD3+ cells in the deep mucosa, some of which are activated by expression of the p55 chain of the IL-2 receptor (CD25) (Fig. 11.2A, 11.2B); (ii) appearance of HLA-DR antigens on crypt enterocytes reflecting a local increase in lymphokine release (IFN-τ) by activated T cells; (iii) a decreased number of Ki67+ proliferating cells within the crypts. Repeated graft biopsies within 24 to 48 hours usually show morphological changes, including crypt necrosis and epithelial damage.

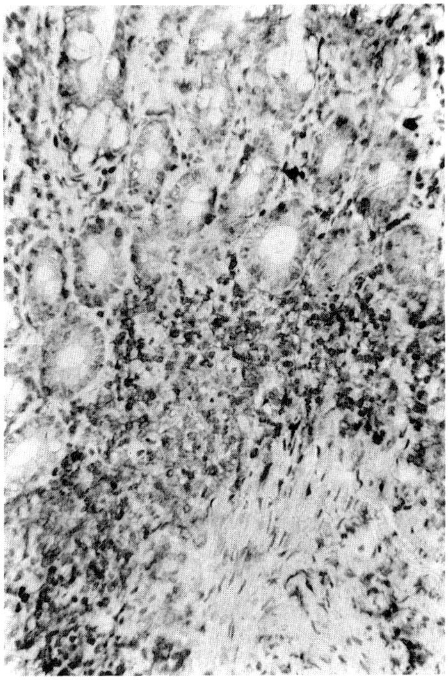

Fig. 11.2a Acute rejection: immunohistochemistry revealed an increased number of CD3+ cells within the lamina propria under the crypts.

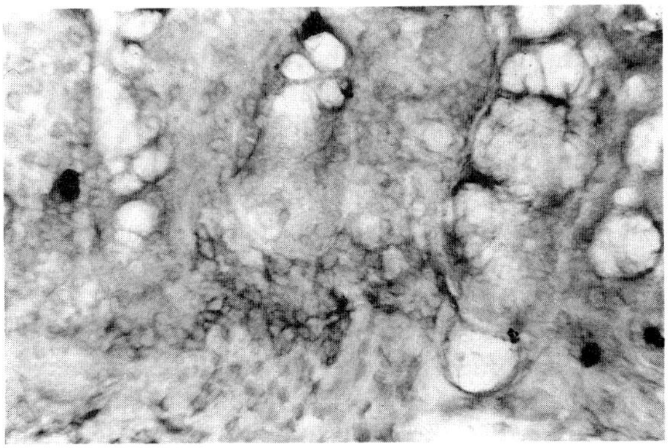

Fig. 11.2b Acute rejection: immunohistochemistry revealed the presence in the lamina propria infiltrate under the crypts of CD25+ lymphoid cells corresponding to activated cells bearing interleukin-2 receptor.

By initiating appropriate and early treatment, rapid and efficient control of the rejection process is obtained with a marked decrease of LP CD3+ lymphocytes within a few days, followed by the reappearance of Ki67+ crypt enterocytes and the progressive disappearance of activated T cells (CD25). Finally, Class II antigen expression by crypt enterocytes also disappears. Nevertheless, in two patients (n°5 and n°7 – Table I and II) who received preventive treatment with antilymphocyte globulin, early changes in immunosuppressive therapy using anti-CD3 monoclonal antibodies did not control acute rejection. Graft removal occurred within the first weeks after small bowel transplantation. In those patients, infiltration of LP by activated T cells and CD68+ macrophages increased rapidly while crypt necrosis became extensive and was associated with blunting of villi and sloughing of surface epithelium. Polymorphonuclear cells accumulated in the mucosal vessels, then extruded into the lamina propria and into the crypt lumen. In the most severe cases, mucosal epithelial structures were almost totally destroyed and replaced by an infiltrate of activated macrophages and polymorphonuclear cells. Hansman et al. suggested that the appearance of numerous CD68+ (KiM6+, KiM7+) macrophages in the submucosa could be interpreted as an early sign of graft rejection.[39] This assessment requires a deep or full-thickness biopsy, which is not feasible in all patients on a daily basis. In our paediatric experience the submucosa was either absent or very small, which prevented the use of this marker.

Graft rejection can occur early, within the first two or three weeks following transplantation, as well as later during the post-transplant course. The most severe episodes of rejection occurred early and sometimes led to graft removal. Nevertheless, like others,[16–19] we also observed delayed acute rejection with similar histological and immunohistological patterns, which responded to increased immunosuppressive therapy.

In all circumstances, early detection of rejection is important in order to adjust immunosuppressive therapy. The pathogenesis of intestinal

mismatched intestinal transplantation. The fate of host and donor lymphocytes was followed in three patients treated with FK 506 after small bowel transplantation, either isolated or combined with the liver.[44] During the first week after transplantation, flow cytometry indicated that 5–11 per cent of the circulating lymphocytes were of donor origin although there were no clinical signs of GVHD. By 12–54 days after transplantation, circulating donor lymphocytes were no longer detected. Progressive replacement of lymphocytes in the lamina propria by those of the recipient HLA phenotype was observed on serial biopsies. While lymphoid re-population was considered complete, the epithelial cells of the mucosa remained of graft origin. Such lymphoid repopulation has already been shown to occur after successful transplantation in piglets.[45]

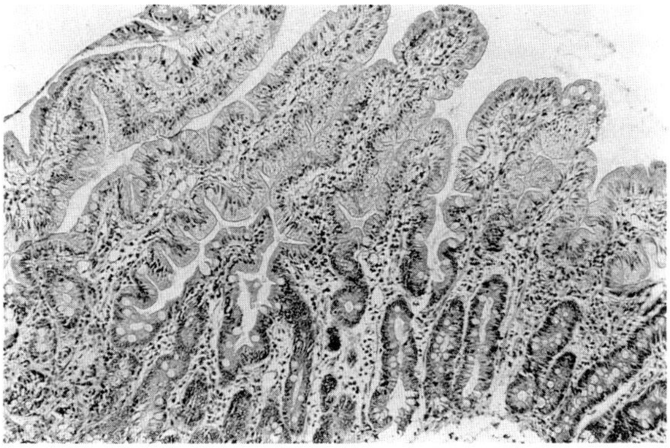

Fig. 11.5 Normal intestinal biopsy 3 years after small bowel transplantation.

Conclusion

Isolated cadaveric small bowel transplantation remains a challenge with severe rejection the major problem despite early and efficient diagnosis and treatment. In our experience, a 5 year-old girl has maintained normal graft function (Fig. 11.5) 4 years after isolated, cadaveric small bowel transplantation. This patient still receives cyclosporin, low-dose steroids, and azathioprine. Recent reports from the transplant programme at Pittsburgh, USA, have demonstrated that the long-term acceptance of isolated small bowel grafts can be achieved using FK 506.[17,19] Clinical and experimental results of combined small bowel/liver transplantation demonstrate the enhancement of small intestine graft survival induced by the liver.[16–19,46–48] Nevertheless, in a model of splanchnic transplantation, Murase et al. failed to demonstrate this protective effect of the liver on the small bowel graft.[49] Small bowel/liver transplantation seems to be most appropriate for patients with anatomical or functional small intestine insufficiency from end-stage liver disease, either related to parenteral nutrition or primitive liver disease. Long-term survival and adaptation of short bowel syndrome after neonatal resection may be achieved by using home parenteral nutrition.[50,51] However, in the near future, patients dependent on total parenteral nutrition[52] should benefit from the further improvements of isolated, cadaveric small bowel transplantation and new immunosuppressive drugs. Whatever the indication and modalities of small bowel transplantation, early diagnosis and treatment of graft rejection will remain an absolute necessity.

References

1. Lillehei RC, Idezulai Y, Feemster JA, et al. Transplantation of stomach, intestine and pancreas: experimental and clinical observations. *Surgery* 1967, **62,** 721–41.
2. Olivier CI, Rettori R, Olivier C. Homotransplantation orthotopique de l'intestin grêle et des côlons droit et transverse chez l'homme. *J Chirurgie (Paris)* 1969; **98,** 323–30.
3. Okumura M, Fujimara I, Ferrari AA. Transplante del intestino delgado, apresentacao de un caso. *Rev Hosp Clin Fac Med San Paolo* 1969; **24,** 39.
4. Alican F, Hardy JD, Cayvili M. Intestine transplantation: laboratory experience and report of a clinical case. *Am J Surg* 1971; **121,** 150–9.
5. Fortner JG, Sichuk G, Litwin SD, Beattie EJ. Immunological response to an intestinal allograft with HLA identical donor-recipient. *Transplantation* 1972; **14,** 531–5.
6. Schraut W. Current status of small bowel transplantation. *Gastroenterology* 1988; **94,** 525–35.
7. Ricour C, Revillon Y, Arnaud-Battandier D, et al. Successful small bowel allografts in piglets using cyclosporine. *Transplant Proc* 1983; **15,** 3109–26.
8. Grant D, Duff J, Zhong R, et al. Successful intestinal transplantation in pigs treated with cyclosporine. *Transplantation* 1988; **45,** 279–84.
9. Saat RE, De Bruin F, Heineman E, Jeekel J, Marquet RL. The limited efficacy of cyclosporine in preventing rejection and graft-versus-host disease in orthotopic small bowel transplantation in rats. *Transplantation* 1990; **50,** 374–7.
10. Masaki Y, Shimazu R, Grogan JB, Subramony C,

Raju S. Histology of host and graft lymphoid tissue in a chronic orthotopic bowel allograft model in the rat. *Transplant Proc* 1991; **23,** 672–4.

11. Watson AJM, Lear PA. Current status of intestinal transplantation. *Gut* 1989; **30,** 1771–82.
12. Starzl TE, Todo S, Tzakis A, Murase N. Multivisceral and intestinal transplantation. *Transplant Proc* 1992; **24,** 1217–23.
13. Cohen Z, Silverman RE, Wassef R. Small intestinal transplantation using cyclosporine. Report of case. *Transplantation* 1986; **42,** 613–21.
14. Schroeder P, Goulet O, Lear P. Small bowel transplantation: European experience. *Lancet* 1990; **336,** 110–11.
15. Goulet O, Revillon Y, Brousse N, et al. Successful small bowel transplantation in an infant. *Transplantation* 1992; **53,** 940–3.
16. Grant D, Wall W, Mimerault R. Successful small bowel–liver transplantation. *Lancet* 1990; **335,** 181–4.
17. Todo S, Tsakis A, Abu-Elmagd K, et al. Cadaveric small bowel and small bowel–liver transplantation in humans. *Transplantation* 1992; **53**(2), 369–76.
18. McAlister V, Wall W, Ghent C, Zhong R, Duff J, Grant D. Successful small intestine transplantation. *Transplant Proc* 1992; **24,** 1236–7.
19. Todo S, Tzakis A, Abu-Elmagd K, et al. Intestinal transplantation in composite visceral grafts or alone. *Ann Surg* 1992; 216, 223.
20. Goulet O, Revillon Y, Jan D, et al. Small bowel transplantation in children. *Transplant Proc* 1990; **22**(6), 2499–500.
21. Nakamura K, Nalesnik M, Jaffe R, Demetris AJ. Morphologic monitoring of human small bowel allografts. *Transplant Proc* 1993; (in press).
22. Ettinger SL, McLoughlin MG, Scudamore CH, Miller RR, Keown PA. Effect of recovery from ischaemic injury on Class I and Class II MHC antigen expression. *Transplantation* 1990; **49,** 641–4.
23. Brousse N, Jarry A, Canioni D, et al. Intestinal transplantation in children: contribution of immunohistochemistry. *Transplant Proc* 1990; **22,** 2495–6.
24. Nordgren S, Cohen Z, MacKenzie R, et al. Functional monitors of rejection in small intestinal transplants. *Am J Surg* 1984; **147,** 152–8.
25. Schraut WH, Lee KK. Monitoring of small bowel allograft rejection maltose absorption. In Deltz E, Thiede A, Hamelmann H (eds) *Small Bowel Transplantation: Experimental and Clinical Fundamentals*. Heidelberg, Springer-Verlag, pp. 241–9, 1985.
26. Silverman R, Cohen Z, Levy G, et al. Immune responses in small intestinal transplantation in the rat: correlation of histopathology and monocyte procoagulant activity. *Surgery* 1987; **102,** 395–402.
27. Meijssen MA, Heineman E, De Bruin RW, Ten Kate FJ, Marquet RL, Molanaar JC. Detection of canine intestinal allograft rejection by *in vivo* electro-physiologic monitoring. *Transplantation* 1991; **51,** 955–9.
28. Grant D, Hurlbut D, Zhong R, et al. Intestinal permeability and bacterial translocation following small bowel transplantation in the rat. *Transplantation* 1991; **52,** 221–4.
29. Schmid T, Oberhuber G, Körözsi G, Klima G, Margreiter R. Histologic pattern of small bowel allograft rejection in the rat. Mucosal biopsies do not provide sufficient information. *Gastroenterology* 1989; **96,** 1529–32.
30. Wallander J, Johnson C, Hällgren R, Gerdin B, Tufveson G. Intestinal distribution and leakage of hyaluroman in small bowel allografting in the rat. *Transplant Proc* 1992; **24,** 1100–1.
31. Maeda K, Schwartz MZ, Bamberger MH, Daniller A. A possible serum marker for rejection after small intestine transplantation. *Am J Surg* 1987; **153,** 68–74.
32. Schroeder P, Gundlach M, Quaroni A, Hansmann ML, Schweizer E, Deltz E. Follow-up of small bowel transplantation by monoclonal antibodies against brush-border membranes. *Transplant Proc* 1990; **22,** 2476.
33. Hansman ML, Deltz E, Gundlach M, Schroeder P, Radzun HJ. Small bowel transplantation in a child. Morphologic, immunohistochemical and clinical results. *Am J Clin Pathol* 1989; **92,** 686–92.
34. Brousse N, Sarnacki S, Canioni D, Cerf-Bensussan N. Immunology of intestinal transplantation in humans and animals. In MacDonald TT (ed.) *Immunology of Gastrointestinal Disease*. London, Kluwer, pp. 87–103, 1992.
35. Schroeder P. Schweizer E, Hansmann ML, et al. Monitoring in small bowel transplantation using cytochemistry and immunochemistry: a comparison of different techniques. *Transplant Proc* 1991; **23,** 675–6.
36. Yamatoka A, Miyano T, Fukunaga K, et al. Patchy distribution of rejection changes in small intestinal transplantation. *J Pediatr Surg* 1992; **27,** 602–3.
37. Wright HI, Abu-Elmagd K, Nakamura K, et al. The role of endoscopy in small bowel transplantation. *Gastroenterology* 1992; **102,** 910 (abstract).
38. Cerf-Bensussan N, Schneeberger EE, Bahn AK. Immunohistologic and immunoelectron microscopic characterisation of the mucosal lymphocytes of human small intestine by the use of monoclonal antibodies. *J Immunol* 1983; **130,** 2615–22.
39. Hansman ML, Hell K, Gundlach M, Deltz E, Schroeder P. Immunohistochemical investigation of biopsies in a successful small bowel transplantation. *Transplant Proc* 1990; **22,** 2502–3.
40. Mowat AMcI. Intestinal graft-*versus*-host disease. In MacDonald TT (ed.) *Immunology of Gastrointestinal Tract*. London, Kluwer, pp. 105–36, 1992.
41. Fromont G, Peuchmaur M, Devergne O, et al.

Small bowel transplantation in children: *in situ* cytokines and serine esterase B gene expression in allograft rejection. *Transplantation* (submitted).
42. Mosnier JF, Cerf-Bensussan N, Calise D, et al. Immunohistochemical study of intestinal allografts in rats. *Proc 1st Int Symp Small Bowel Transplant.* October 10–13, 1989, London, England.
43. MacDonald TT, Ferguson A. Hypersensitivity reactions in small intestine III. The effect of allograft rejection and of graft-*versus*-host disease on epithelial cell kinetics. *Cell Tissue Kinet* 1977; **10,** 301–12.
44. Iwaki Y, Starzl IE, Yagihasni A, et al. Replacement of donor lymphoid tissue in small bowel transplants. *Lancet* 1991; **337,** 818–19.
45. Arnaud-Battandier F, Salmon H, Vaiman M, et al. Small intestinal transplantation in swine with cyclosporine treatment: studies of intestinal lymphoid populations. *Transplant Proc* 1985; **17,** 1440–1.
46. Sarnacki S, Revillon Y, Cerf-Bensussan N, Calise D, Goulet O, Brousse N. Long-term small bowel graft survival induced by spontaneously tolerated liver allograft in inbred rat strains. *Transplantation* (in press).
47. Li X, Zhong R, He G, et al. Host immunosuppression after combined liver/intestine transplantation in the rat. *Transplant Proc* 1992; **24,** 1206–7.
48. Zhong R, He G, Sakai Y et al. The effect of donor –recipient strain combinations in combined liver/intestine transplantation in the rat. *Transplant Proc* 1992; **24,** 1208–9.
49. Murase N, Demetris AJ, Kim GD, et al. Rejection of the multivisceral allografts in rats: a sequential analysis with comparison to isolated orthotopic, small bowel and liver grafts. *Surgery* 1990; **108,** 880–9.
50. Goulet O, Revillon Y, Jan D et al. Neonatal short bowel syndrome. *J Pediatr* 1991; **119**(1), 18–23.
51. Ricour C, Gorski AM, Goulet O, et al. Home parenteral nutrition in children: eight years of experience with 112 patients. *Hum Nutr Clin Nutr* 1990; **9,** 65–71.
52. Goulet O, Revillon Y, Jan D, et al. Which patients need small bowel transplantation for neonatal short bowel syndrome. *Transplant Proc* 1992; **24,** 1058–9.

12

Clinical small bowel transplantation

Vivian C McAlister and David R Grant

Those who cannot remember the past are condemned to repeat it.

George Santayana

Overview

Pioneering studies by Alexis Carrel at the turn of this century demonstrated the technical feasibility of intestinal transplantation and correctly predicted that the main hurdle to this operation would be the control of rejection.[1,2] Small bowel transplantation was first attempted in humans in the early 1960s. Parenteral nutrition was not available at that time and physicians were haunted by the spectre of young, previously healthy patients dying of starvation after massive small bowel resections. The early reports of successful kidney grafting[3] and the perfection of the surgical techniques for small bowel transplantation in dogs by Lillehei and colleagues[4] provided further impetus for this procedure.

The first intestinal recipients were treated with steroids, antilymphocyte globulin, and azathioprine. None survived. In retrospect, these cases were probably doomed to failure from the outset because of the poor understanding of the immunology of small bowel grafting at that time. As Starzl has commented: 'The intestinal baby was premature and remained ICU-bound for thirty years.'[5]

The early 1980s witnessed significant advancement in our understanding of intestinal preservation; perioperative care; the immunology of small bowel transplantation; the detection and prevention of intestinal rejection; and the physiology of the small bowel graft.[6] Armed with this knowledge, the first successful clinical small bowel transplants were performed in the late 1980s.[7,9] At the time of writing this chapter, approximately 40 intestinal recipients have been able to stop total parenteral nutrition (TPN) and resume normal lives.

Isolated small intestinal transplantation using conventional immunosuppression

The first successful kidney transplant was performed between identical twins in 1954.[10] Inroads into monitoring and controlling rejection soon permitted allotransplantation using azathioprine and steroids.[11,12] Early work with antilymphocyte sera marked the beginning of a search for stronger immunosuppressive agents.[13–15] It was in this setting that the clinical application of intestinal transplantation began (Table 12.1), borrowing elements of both surgical technique and immunosuppression from renal transplantation.

The first two cases of intestinal transplantation were performed by Deterling and colleagues at the Boston Floating Hospital in 1964.[16] Unfortunately, neither of these cases have been reported in detail. In the first procedure, a segment of ileum was transplanted from a mother to her child. A cadaveric intestinal graft was transplanted into a second child later that year. Both grafts infarcted soon after the transplant surgery and were removed.

The next reported transplant was performed by Lillehei and associates in 1967 using the small intestine and ascending colon from a cadaveric donor.[17] The recipient's intestine had previously been resected for gangrene due to portal and mesenteric venous thrombosis. The graft was placed heterotopically with vascular anastomoses to the

Table 12.1 Isolated small intestine transplantation before cyclosporin

Year	Centre	Graft	Transplanted	Outcome (graft survival)
1964	Boston	segment ileum	Mother to child	Graft necrosis (12 hours)[16]
1964	Boston	SI	Cadaver to child	Graft necrosis (2 days)[16]
1967	Minnesota	SI and colon	Cadaver to adult	Graft necrosis (12 hours)[17]
1968	Sao Paulo	SI	Cadaver to adult	Graft necrosis (10 days)[18]
1969	Paris	SI/right colon	Cadaver to adult	Rejection (26 days)[20]
1969	Jackson, Mississippi	ileum 100 cm	Mother to child	Graft necrosis (7 days)[22]
1970	Sao Paulo	SI	Cadaver to child	Graft necrosis (5 days)[19]
1970	New York	ileum 170 cm	Sister to adult*	Died sepsis (76 days)[23,24]

Abbreviations: SI – entire small intestine
*HLA identical

recipient's iliac artery and vein. Each end of the intestine was exteriorized as a stoma. The graft thrombosed within 12 hours and the patient died.

Okumura in Brazil achieved a 10-day patient survival in a 34 year-old female using this same technique of surgical reconstruction in 1968.[18] The graft had been removed from the donor during open cardiac massage. The recipient's intestine had been resected because of a thrombosis of the superior mesenteric artery. On reperfusion, cyanotic segments of the graft were excised. The two stomata appeared dusky on several occasions during the postoperative period and they were trimmed. The graft was removed on the tenth postoperative day because of total necrosis. The patient died on the twelfth postoperative day. Okumura performed a second cadaveric transplant on a 12 year-old girl in 1970.[19] The graft thrombosed on the fifth postoperative day. Reviewing these cases, it is impossible to determine if the graft loss was due to a technical complication or acute rejection.

The fifth attempt at intestinal transplantation was made by Olivier and colleagues in Paris, France in 1969.[20,21] This patient was the first of many to undergo small bowel transplantation for Gardner's syndrome and a mesenteric desmoid tumour. This patient received an HLA-mismatched cadaveric graft of the entire intestine and right colon. Proximal enteric continuity was restored. Immunosuppression included antilymphocyte serum, azathioprine, and steroids. The graft and the patient did well until the tenth postoperative day when diarrhoea and abdominal distention developed as a result of rejection. Switching from azathioprine to 6-mercaptopurine failed to halt this process. The patient died on the twenty-sixth postoperative day. Post-mortem examination revealed patchy, full-thickness necrosis of the intestine with an intense mononuclear cell infiltrate and patent large vessels. This was the first case report of the clinical and pathological features of intestinal rejection.

In 1969, Alican and associates from the University of Mississippi performed a living-related transplant in a 10 year-old boy who had lost his entire small bowel to a strangulating mesenteric band.[22] A segment of ileum (100 cm) was removed from the child's mother and then transplanted heterotopically. The graft was removed on the seventh postoperative day because of necrosis. Pathological examination revealed minimal inflammation of the graft. Again, it is difficult to tell in retrospect whether the graft loss was due to a technical complication or rejection, but the former diagnosis seems more likely in view of the pathological findings.

Fortner and colleagues transplanted a 170 cm segment of ileum from a sibling into a 37 year-old woman with Gardner's syndrome in 1970.[23,24] The patient had been maintained on TPN for 16 months prior to transplantation. HLA identity was established based on the typing sera available at that time and a negative mixed lymphocyte culture. The hypogastric artery and external iliac vein were used to revascularize the graft. Enteric continuity at both proximal and distal ends was restored. An isolated pouch of ileum was brought out to the skin to provide access for mucosal biopsies to monitor for rejection. Immunosuppression included antilymphocyte serum and azathioprine. On the nineteenth postoperative day, mucosal changes in the pouch were interpreted as rejection. The patient was treated with steroids and the histological abnormalities were resolved. She started eating on the twenty-third day and tolerated a normal diet although TPN was continued. During the second month, the patient de veloped recurrent bacterial and fungal sepsis. She died in septic shock on the seventy-fifth postoperative day. At autopsy no source of infection was found. The graft was mildly atrophic. Histology revealed minor flattening of the villi with maintenance of the crypts. There was no clear evidence of rejection.

Isolated small intestinal transplantation using cyclosporin

Interest in small bowel transplantation waned in the late 1960s after the introduction of total parenteral nutrition. Interest was revived a decade later when the limitations of TPN were becoming more evident and cyclosporin was being successfully used for clinical heart and liver transplantation.

Cyclosporin was first tried after small bowel transplantation by Cohen and associates of Toronto, Canada in 1985 (Table 12.2).[25] A blood group O cadaveric graft was transplanted into a 26 year-old, blood group A woman with Gardner's syndrome. This patient's entire small intestine had been resected a year earlier because of a large desmoid tumour. The superior mesenteric artery was anastomosed to the aorta; the superior mesenteric vein was drained into the inferior vena cava. The ends of the intestine were exteriorized. Immunosuppression included parenteral cyclosporin, 4–9 mg/kg/day, and methylprednisolone tapered to 20 mg/day by the sixth day. On the fourth postoperative day, a severe haemolytic anaemia developed in association with high titres of anti-A antibodies. On the ninth postoperative day, the recipient suddenly became comatose. The graft was removed the following day. It appeared grossly normal. Histological examination revealed early rejection with a moderate mononuclear infiltrate and preservation of the intestinal villi. The recipient's neurological condition never improved. She died on the eleventh postoperative day. Autopsy revealed an unexplained thalamic infarction.

Williams and colleagues performed a small intestine transplant in a 14 year-old girl whose small bowel had been removed because of a gunshot injury.[26] A non-HLA-matched, crossmatch negative cadaveric donor was used. A cobalt-60 source delivered 1750 rad to the *ex vivo* graft. The small bowel was implanted in a heterotopic location. The patient was treated with intravenous cyclosporin, 7 mg/kg/day, and methylprednisolone, 1.5 mg/kg/day in tapering doses. The stomas appeared dark on the third postoperative day. Biopsies showed acute rejection which was successfully abrogated with high-dose steroids. On

Table 12.2 Isolated small intestine transplantation with cyclosporin

Year	Centre	Immunosuppression	Transplanted	Outcome (graft survival)
1985	Toronto	CyA-Ster	Cadaver to adult*	Hemolysis, come (11 days)[25]
1987	Chicago	CyA-Ster	Cadaver to child	Rejection (10 days)[26]
1987	Paris	CyA-Ster	Cadaver to infant**	Thrombosis (3 hours)[9,28]
1987	Paris	CyA-Ster	Cadaver to child	Liver/renal failure (6 months)[27]
1987	Kiel	CyA-Ster-ATG	Mother to child	Rejection (12 days)[31]
1988	London (Ontario)	CyA-Ster-Aza-ALG	Cadaver to child†	Rejection (14 days)[30]
1988	Kiel	CyA-Ster-ATG	Half-sister to adult††	TPN free, Lymphoma, alive[8]
1988	Paris	CyA-Ster-ALG	Cadaver to child	Chronic rejection (17 months)[9,28]
1989	Paris	CyA-Ster-Aza-ALG	Cadaver to child**	Rejection/removed (2 months)[9,28]
1989	Paris	CyA-Ster-Aza-ALG	Cadaver to infant	TPN free, alive[9,28]
1989	Uppsala	CyA-Ster-Aza-ALG	Cadaver to child	Rejection, sepsis (56 days)[34]
1990	Paris	CyA-Ster-Aza-ALG	Cadaver to infant*	Hemolysis, rejection (21 days)[28,71]
1990	Paris	CyA-Ster-Aza-ALG	Cadaver to child	Perioperative shock[9]

Abbreviations: CyA-cyclosporin; Ster-steroids; Aza-azathioprine; ALG-antilymphocyte globulin; ATG-antithymocyte globulin; TPN-total parenteral nutrition

*ABO mismatch, O to A; **same recipient, retransplanted 2 years later; † OKT3 and ALG donor pretreatment; ††partial HLA match.

Table 12.4 Clinical intestinal transplantation at the University of Pittsburgh – overall experience

Pt.	Age	Sex	Indication	Type of intestinal graft	Survival* Patient	Survival* Graft	Current status
1	31	M	Gunshot wound	Intestine	25.5	21.9	Graft removed, retransplant
				Intestine		2.3	Died, sepsis
2	3.2	F	Necrotizing enterocolitis	Intestine – Liver	>35.9	>35.9	TPN – Free
3	26	F	SMA thrombosis	Intestine – Liver	>35.5	>35.5	TPN – Free
4	4.3	M	Gastroschisis	Intestine – Liver	>31.8	>31.8	TPN – Free
5	2.8	M	Intestinal atresia	Intestine – Liver	12.6	12.6	Died, PTLD
6	0.6	F	Intestinal atresia	Intestine – Liver	0.8	0.8	Died, sepsis and ? GVHD
7	1.1	F	Volvulus	Intestine – Liver	>23.3	>23.3	TPN – Free
8	1.7	F	Volvulus	Intestine – Liver	>23.3	>23.3	TPN – Free
9	21	M	Traffic accident	Intestine – Liver	>23.0	>23.0	TPN – Partial
10	32	M	CA & SMA thrombosis	Multivisceral	>21.2	>21.2	TPN – Free
11	2.5	F	Microvillus inclusion disease	Intestine	>20.6	>20.6	TPN – Free
12	1.3	M	Intestinal atresia	Intestine	>18.8	>18.8	TPN – Free
13	50	F	Crohn's disease	Intestine	>18.7	>18.7	TPN – Free
14	34	F	Desmoid tumour	Intestine	14.5	7.9	Graft removed, died
15	38	M	Crohn's disease	Intestine	12.4	12.0	Died, sepsis and liver failure
16	10.2	F	Pseudo-obstruction	Intestine	>16.5	>16.5	TPN – partial
17	22	F	Crohn's disease	Intestine	>16.3	>16.3	TPN – Free
18	25	M	Crohn's disease	Intestine – Liver	>15.7	>15.7	TPN – Free
19	1.5	M	Necrotizing enterocolitis	Intestine – Liver	2.3	2.3	Died, MOF and sepsis
20	29	F	Desmoid tumor	Intestine – Liver	>13.8	>13.8	TPN – Free
21	24	M	CA & SMA thrombosis	Multivisceral	>13.7	>13.7	TPN – Free
22	20	F	Traffic accident	Intestine	>13.4	>13.4	TPN – Free
23	4.2	F	Gastroschisis	Intestine – Liver	>13.3	>13.3	TPN – Free
24	1.4	M	Gastroschisis	Intestine – Liver	1.0	1.0	Died, sepsis
25	0.75	M	Microvillus inclusion disease	Intestine – liver	>12.0	>12.0	TPN – Free
26	0.5	M	Gastroschisis	Intestine – Liver	>11.8	>11.8	TPN – Free
27	31	F	CA & SMA thrombosis	Multivisceral	>11.3	>11.3	TPN – Free
28	19.1	M	Traffic accident	Intestine – Liver	>11.2	>11.2	TPN – Free
29	44	F	SMA thrombosis	Intestine – Liver	>10.4	>10.4	TPN – Free
30	4.5	F	Pseudo-obstruction	Multivisceral	> 8.5	> 8.5	TPN – Free
31	42	F	Budd-Chiari	Multivisceral			Died – Intraoperative bleeding, pre-TX
32	37	F	Familial polyposis	Intestine	> 7.7	> 7.7	TPN – Free
33	3.6	M	Necrotizing enterocolitis	Intestine – Liver	3.5	2.0	Retransplanted, rejection
				Intestine – Liver		1.5	Died, rejection
34	0.87	F	Gastroschisis	Intestine – Liver	> 7.2	> 7.2	TPN – Free
35	15.5	M	Volvulus	Intestine – Liver	> 6.5	> 6.6	TPN – Free
36	44	M	Gastrinoma	Multivisceral	1.6	1.6	Died – pneumonia, ARDS
37	28	M	Alpha-1-antitrypsin	Multivisceral			Died – intraoperative PE, pre-TX
38	39	M	Crohn's disease	Intestine	> 5.1	> 5.1	TPN – Free
39	35.5	M	Crohn's disease	Intestine	4.0	4.0	Died, respiratory distress
40	58.0	F	Resection for colon CA	Intestine	> 4.6	> 4.6	TPN – Free
41	3.0	F	Necrotizing enterocolitis	Intestine – Liver	0.9	0.9	Died, pneumonia
42	1.7	M	Gastroschisis	Intestine	> 4.1	0.9	Graft removed, ALIVE
43	1.8	F	Multiple polyposis	Modified multivisceral**	> 4.0	> 4.0	TPN – Free
44	9.6	M	Volvulus	Intestine	> 3.7	> 3.7	TPN – Free
45	32.6	M	Budd-Chiari	Multivisceral	> 3.2	> 3.2	TPN – Free
46	3.6	F	Volvulus	Intestine – Liver	> 2.1	> 2.1	TPN – Free
47	0.8	F	Jejunal atresia	Intestine – Liver	> 1.9	> 1.9	TPN – Free
48	10.9	F	Pseudo-obstruction	Multivisceral	> 1.8	> 1.8	TPN – Free
49	1.7	F	Necrotizing enterocolitis	Intestine – Liver	1.0	1.0	Died – sepsis, GVHD
50	34.1	M	Crohn's disease	Intestine	0.7	0.7	Died – seizure CA
51	3.4	M	Volvulus	Intestine – Liver	> 1.6	> 1.6	TPN – Partial
52	1.3	F	Hirshsprung's disease	Intestine – Liver	> 1.0	> 1.0	TPN – Partial
53	50.0	F	Intestinal adhesions	Intestine	> 0.5	> 0.5	TPN – Partial

Abbreviations: SMA-superior mesenteric artery; CA-cancer; TPN-total parenteral nutrition; PTLD-post-transplant lymphoproliferative disease; GVHD-graft-versus-host disease; MOF-multi-organ failure; ARDS-acute respiratory distress syndrome; PE-pulmonary embolism

*Survival in months; **consists of stomach, small bowel, pancreas, and large bowel

cyclosporin era[23] and for the first successful isolated small bowel transplant using cyclosporin.[8] However, it is of note that the latter recipient still had 5 rejection episodes requiring recurrent treatment with steroids and antithymocyte globulin.

Donor pretreatment

Experimental studies have shown that donor pretreatment with antilymphocyte agents and/or graft radiation reduces the incidence of graft-versus-host disease (GVHD) but not of rejection.[53,54] The role of donor pretreatment for clinical small bowel transplantation is still controversial. The benefits are unproven and pretreatment may contribute to postoperative lymphomas.

Graft preservation

Most centres have treated the donors with oral and intravenous antibiotics. Bowel preparation with osmotic agents has generally been avoided as the graft becomes difficult to handle when it contains large quantities of entrapped fluid.

Perfusion and storage of intestinal grafts with the University of Wisconsin solution have permitted cold ischaemia times of up to 10 hours with satisfactory graft function.[50] Storage for 16 hours in a case led to the demise of the patient due to graft necrosis and the development of multiple organ failure.[55] Data from pancreatic preservation have suggested that perfusion of non-hepatic viscera should be restricted to less than one litre.[47] If necessary, the liver can be separately perfused via a catheter in the inferior mesenteric vein.[56]

Vascular reconstruction

Portal venous drainage of the small bowel allows the liver to filter translocated organisms and toxins,[57] provides nutrients to the liver,[58] and confers a slight immunological advantage to the graft.[59,60] It is controversial whether these advantages justify the increased technical complexity, which anastomosis to the portal venous system requires, when compared with the easier anastomosis to the vena cava. Various methods have been used for successful arterial reconstruction of the small bowel graft.[39] A conduit of donor thoracic aorta and upper abdominal aorta containing the origins of the celiac and superior mesenteric arteries can be rotated for anastomosis to the recipient's infra-renal aorta, thereby preserving the origins of the donor renal arteries.[7] The donor abdominal aorta can also be used when the inferior mesenteric artery and left colon are transplanted as part of the graft.[39]

Gastrointestinal reconstruction

The proximal end of the intestinal graft has been joined to the native intestine in many cases with a low rate of anastomotic leakage. Early restoration of intestinal continuity is theoretically desirable as it provides potential benefits for graft barrier function and mucosal regeneration.[61] The use of isolated pouches or defunctioned chimneys for surveillance may not accurately reflect the status of an in-continuity intestinal graft since the defunctioned intestine tends to atrophy. The safety of the distal intestinal anastomosis depends on the quality of blood supply to the remaining native intestine. Distal continuity may improve fluid absorption, but it also restricts easy access to the graft for mucosal biopsies to monitor for rejection during the high-risk postoperative period.

Graft-versus-host disease (GVHD)

The overt clinical syndrome of GVHD that is frequently seen after bone marrow transplantation has not been reported after small intestine transplantation in humans. One of the small intestine/liver recipients had a transient erythematous rash which coincided with the appearance of donor lymphocytes in the peripheral circulation. However, this rash settled in 2 days without increasing immunosuppression.[7] Iwaki and colleagues have reported the routine transient appearance of donor lymphocytes in the recipient's circulation without clinical evidence of GVHD[62] and suggested that functioning donor lymphocytes are required for normal cell traffic and lymphocyte replacement after small bowel transplantation.[62] Cytokines, released by the mixed lymphocyte reaction taking place after transplantation, may explain why some patients appear toxic several days after small bowel grafting.

Rejection

Rejection starts as a patchy process and rapidly progresses to full-thickness graft necrosis.[20,30] The incidence and severity of rejection appears to be less in patients with simultaneous liver grafts.[44,51] The transplanted intestinal mucosa can be denuded by severe rejection and still regenerate.[8,27]

Better methods are needed to detect early intestinal rejection. Routine histological examination of mucosal biopsies is subject to sampling error and difficulties in interpretation due to nonspecific inflammation at the stomata and in the defunctioned bowel. The sensitivity of mucosal biopsies for the detection of rejection may be increased by using electron microscopy or immunohistochemical techniques.[63,64] Measurement of graft barrier function is one method of screening the entire graft for rejection but a positive result is not specific for rejection. Cohen and associates found measurement of procoagulant factor helpful for the detection of rejection after experimental transplantation and in their single case of human intestinal transplantation.[25]

Sepsis

Frequent bacterial, fungal, and viral infections have been reported by every small intestine transplant programme. Prevention of graft rejection requires a high degree of immunosuppression and this has undoubtedly contributed to frequent postoperative sepsis. Small bowel/liver recipients appear to have a particularly high risk of sepsis and these combined grafts may require less immunosuppression than other solid organ transplants.

Translocation of organisms across the gut is another factor that has been implicated as a possible source of sepsis after small bowel transplantation. Early enteral feeding may help to optimize gut barrier function.[61] Long-term use of broad spectrum antibiotics and selective bowel decontamination do not appear to prevent sepsis after small bowel grafting.[28,65]

Lymphoma

There has been a very high incidence of lymphomas after small bowel transplantation. Where it has been studied, the lymphomas were associated with the Epstein–Barr virus and were composed of cells of recipient origin.[40,66] Patients with multivisceral grafts appear to have a particularly high risk, possibly because of the large mass of transplanted lymphoid tissue. Intense, nonspecific immunosuppression and donor pretreatment with antilymphocyte products may predispose patients to this complication. Potential measures to reduce the risk of postoperative lymphomas include 1) using as little immunosuppression as possible, 2) prophylactic treatment with gamma globulin containing high titres of anti-EBV antibodies, and 3) prophylactic treatment with Acyclovir.®

Graft function

Successful intestinal transplantation restores grossly normal gut function. Animal studies have shown that transplantation and denervation of the intestine adversely affects carbohydrate and fat absorption, chloride secretion, and specific IgA secretion[67–69] but these problems have not been apparent in human recipients. Gut barrier function appears to return to normal by the fifth postoperative day.[7] Enteral feeding can be introduced in the first week after transplantation[34,44] and TPN can usually be stopped by the second month.[44,51] D-xylose and fat excretion may be abnormal for up to 6 months but they usually return to normal range.[44] Vitamin B_{12} absorption is normal. Crude estimates of small intestine motility have shown normal patterns of peristalsis and transit.[70] The gradual resumption of oral diets in the longest-surviving patients in Paris, France and Kiel, Germany suggests that transplanted bowel is capable of adaptation, similar to normal bowel. Colon transplantation, as suggested by K. Jeejeebhoy in Chapter 1, is a potential method to improve the function of the small bowel graft.

Summary

Until recently, the history of clinical small intestinal transplantation has been marked by failure, despite technical expertise by surgeons and heroism by patients and their families. However, significant progress has occurred in the last 3 years. Combined small bowel/liver grafting has proven to be a feasible treatment for patients who have developed liver failure on TPN. Isolated intestinal grafting with FK506 has become a viable alternative to TPN for the treatment of the short gut syndrome.

References

1. Carrel A. La technique operatoire des anastomoses vasculaires et la transplantation des visceres. *Lyon MEO* 1902; **98,** 859.
2. Carrel A. The transplantation of organs. A preliminary communication. *JAMA* 1905; **45,** 1654.
3. Hume DM, Merrill JP. Miller BF, Thorn GW. Experience in renal homotransplantation in the human: Report of nine cases. *J Clin Invest* 1955; **34,** 327.

4. Lillehei RC, Goott B, Miller FA. The physiological response of the small bowel of the dog to ischemia including prolonged in vitro preservation of the bowel with successful replacement and survival. *Ann Surg* 1959; **150,** 543.
5. Starzl TE, Todo S, Tzakis A, Murase N. Multivisceral and intestinal transplantation. *Transplant Proc* 1992; **24,** 1217.
6. Grant D. Intestinal transplantation: Current status. *Transplant Proc* 1989; **21,** 2869.
7. Grant D, Wall W, Mimeault R, et al. Successful small-bowel/liver transplantation. *Lancet* 1990; **335,** 181.
8. Deltz E, Schroeder, P, Gundlach M, Hansmann ML, Leimenstoll G. Successful clinical small-bowel transplantation. *Transplant Proc* 1990; **22,** 2501.
9. Revillon Y, Jan D, Goulet O, Ricour C. Small bowel transplantation in seven children: preservation technique. *Transplant Proc* 1991; **23,** 2350.
10. Merrill JP, Murray JE, Harrison JH, et al. Successful homotransplant of a human kidney between identical twins. *JAMA* 1956; **160,** 277.
11. Starzl TE, Marchioro TL, Waddell WR. The reversal of rejection in human renal homograft with subsequent development of homograft tolerance. *Surg Gynecol Obstet* 1963; **117,** 385.
12. Murray JE, Harrison JH. Surgical management of fifty patients with kidney transplant including eighteen pairs of twins. *Am J Surg* 1963; **105,** 205.
13. Woodruff MFA, Forman B. Effect of antilymphocyte serum on suspensions of lymphocytes in vitro. *Nature* 1951; **168,** 35.
14. Russell PS, Monaco AP. Heterologous antilymphocyte sera and some of their effects. *Transplantation* 1967; **5,** suppl, 1086.
15. Monaco AP, Wood ML, Russell PS. Effect of adult thymectomy on the recovery from immunological depression induced by anti-lymphocyte serum. *Surg Forum* 1965; **16,** 209.
16. Deterling R. Discussion of paper by Alican F, Hardy JD, Cayirili M, et al. Intestinal transplantation: laboratory experience and a report of a clinical case. *Am J Surg* 1971; **121,** 150.
17. Lillehei RC, Idezuki Y, Feemster JA, et al. Transplantation of stomach, intestine, and pancreas: experimental and clinical observations. *Surgery* 1967; **62,** 721.
18. Okumura M, Fujimura I, Ferrari AA, et al. Transplante de intestino delgado. Apresentacao de um caso. *Rev Hosp Clin Fac Med Sao Paulo* 1969; **24,** 39.
19. Okumura M, Mester M. The coming of age of small bowel transplantation: a historical perspective. *Transplant Proc* 1992; **24,** 1241.
20. Olivier C, Rettori R, Camilleri JP. Interruption of the lymphatic vessels and its consequences in total homotransplantation of the small intestine and right side of the colon in man. *Lymphology* 1972; **5,** 24.
21. Olivier CL, Retorri R, Olivier CH, et al. Homotransplantation orthotopique de l'intestin grele et des colons droit et transverse chez l'homme. *J Chir (Paris)* 1969; **98,** 323.
22. Alican F, Hardy JD, Cayirli M, et al. Intestinal transplantation: laboratory experience and report of a clinical case. *Am J Surg* 1971; **121,** 150.
23. Fortner JG, Shiu MH, Kunlin A, et al. Orthotopic intestinal allografting after massive intestinal resection. *Bull la Soc Inter Chir* 1972; **4,** 1.
24. Fortner JG, Sichuk G, Litwin SD, Beattie EJ. Immunological responses to an intestinal allograft with HLA identical donor-recipient. *Transplantation* 1972; **14,** 531.
25. Cohen Z, Silverman RE, Wassef R, et al. Small intestinal transplantation using cyclosporine. Report of a case. *Transplantation* 1986; **42,** 613.
26. Tattersall C, Gebel H, Haklin M, Hartsell W, Williams J. Lymphocyte responsiveness after irradiation in canine and human intestinal allografts. *Curr Surg* 1989; **46,** 16.
27. Goulet OJ, Revillon Y, Cerf-Bensussan N, et al. Small intestinal transplantation in a child using cyclosporine. *Transplant Proc* 1988; **20,** 288.
28. Goulet O, Revillon Y, Jan D, et al. Small-bowel transplantation in children. *Transplant Proc* 1990; **22,** 2499.
29. Grant D, Duff J, Zhong R, et al. Successful intestinal transplantation in pigs treated with cyclosporine. *Transplantation* 1988; **45,** 279.
30. Grant D, Sommerauer J, Mimeault R, et al. Treatment with continuous high dose intraveous cyclosporine following intestinal transplantation. A case report. *Transplantation* 1989; **48,** 151.
31. Hansmann ML, Deltz E, Gundlach M, Schroeder P, Radzun HJ. Small bowel transplantation in a child. *Am J Clin Pathol* 1989; **920,** 686.
32. Deltz E, Mengel W, Hamelmann H. Small bowel transplantation: report of a clinical case. *Prog Pediatr Surg* 1990; **25,** 90.
33. Deltz E. Personal communication. 1992 (unpublished).
34. Wallander J, Ewald U, Lackgren G, Tufveson G, Wahlberg J, Meurling S. Extreme short bowel syndrome in neonates: an indication for small bowel transplantation? *Transplant Proc* 1992; **24,** 1230.
35. Starzl TE, Kaupp HA Jr, Brock DR, Butz GW Jr, Linman JW. Homotransplantation of multiple visceral organs. *Am J Surg* 1962; **103,** 219.
36. Lillehei RC, Idezuki Y, Feemster JA, et al. Transplantation of stomach, intestine and pancreas: experimental and clinical observations. *Surgery* 1967; **62,** 721.
37. Starzl TE, Shaw BW Jr, Nalesnik MA, Hakala TR. Pancreaticoduodenal transplantation in humans. *Surg Gynecol Obstet* 1984; **159,** 265.
38. Starzl TE, Todo S, Tzakis A, et al. Abdominal organ cluster transplantation for the treatment of

Enzymes in intestine 19
Epstein-Barr virus 129
Escherichia coli endotoxin 62, 66
Ethylenediaminetetra-acetate (EDTA) 58
  in diagnosis of rejection 33
Experimental models
  bacterial translocation 61
  cost of 12
  immunosuppression 78–87
  intestinal transplants 9–17, 102
  intestine/liver transplant 106
  motility 25
  on long-term sequelae 15
  physiology of transplants 20
  rejection 12, 13, 14
  transplant function 12
  venous drainage 12, 104

FK 506 14, 88, 101, 112, 126–7, 133
  compared with cyclosporin 38, 82
  effect on allograft survival 82, 83
  immunosuppression 108
  pretreatment with 93, 96
  treatment of recipients 82
FK binding protein 82
Fat
  absorption in transplant 24
  digestion in intestine 19
  measurement of 24
Fatty acids in colon 2
Fluid absorption
  effect of resection on 2
Food allergy 53

Gardner's syndrome 122, 123
Gastric emptying 1
Gastric hypersecretion
  intestinal resection causing 3
Gastric motility 2
Gastrointestinal physiology 1–2, 19
Gastrointestinal reconstruction 128
Glucose absorption in graft 23
Glutamine in preservation 73
Gluten 59
Graft
  bacterial translocation in 65
  cellular infiltration in 32
  combined 101
  cooling of 71
  effect of preservation on histology 113
  isolated 101
  multivisceral 101
  pretreatment *See Pretreatment*
  rejection *See Rejection*
Graft antigens
  contact with host antigens 30
Graft barrier enhancement 66
Graft barrier function 63
Graft cell
  migration to host 35
Graft function 129
  monitoring 20
Graft lymphocytes
  reducing 38
Graft permeability 65
Graft-versus-host disease 10, 11, 30–42, 78, 88, 107, 116, 128
  in animal models 36
  basic conditions 34
  biopsy 117
  development of 13
  diagnosis of 37
  equilibrium with rejection 34, 39
  experimental models 12, 13
  irradiation preventing 38, 79
  leukocytes in 90
  mesenteric lymphadenectomy preventing 93
  pathology of 117
  pretreatment of donor preventing 38, 128
  prevention of 37, 90
Gruenhagen's space 58, 63
Gut-associated lymphoid tissues 57

Haemolytic anaemia 123, 126
Haemorrhagic shock 60
Heterotopic grafts 10, 20
Home parenteral nutrition 5–6, 118
  complications of 6
Host
  graft cell migration to 35
Host antigens
  contact with graft antigens 30
Host cells
  infiltrating graft 32
Host defence system 43
Host lymphocytes
  in donor bowel 51
Host sensitization 30
Host-versus-graft reaction 78
Hyperoxalauria 3
Hypochlorhydria
  neonatal 55
Hypomagnesemia 4
Hypotension 62, 126
Hypothermia
  preservation and 71

Ileal resection 5
  cholelithiasis after 3
Ileum
  electrolyte absorption in 1
  functions of 2
  transplant 122
Immune response 43
Immunogenicity of small bowel 89
Immunoglobulin A 44

deficiency of 44
effect on bacteria 61
in mucosa 57
in mucosal barrier 54
production of 51
production by allografts 45
protective function 44
response to immunization 46
response against T cell independent antigen 50
synthesis 44
total production 45
Immunologic reactions after transplant 12
Immunosuppression 9, 78–87, 121
See also under agents concerned
chemotherapy and 61
combined treatment 92
effect on rejection 32
future prospects 133
increase in GVHD 38
species differences 81
triple-combination therapy 81
Immunosuppressive agents
See also specific drugs
effectiveness of 14
Immunotoxin perfusion 94
Implications for protocols 127
Inferior vena cava
drainage into 102, 105
Inter-digestive myoelectric complex 26
Interleukin-1, -2, -6 30, 82, 83
Intestinal failure 1–8
definition of 1
home parenteral nutrition for 5
transplantation in 6
Intestinal hypertrophy
after resection 25
Intestinal ischaemia 58, 63
lesions following 70
pathophysiology 70
preservation and 70
Intestinal permeability 57–60
abnormalities of 59
definition of 57, 58
endotoxin affecting 62
testing 58
Intestinal resection
complications of 3
effects of 2
hypertrophy following 25
massive 5, 25
nutritional treatment following 3–5
special considerations 5
Intestinal transplantation 6
clinical features 103, 121–32
composite 125
experimental models 9–17
phsiology of 18–29
future of 133
historical cases 104–5
methods of 101
pathology of 112–20
Intestine
adaptation 24
growth and metabolism after transplant 24
immune response 43
normal absorption 19
normal digestion 19
resident flora 56
role of enzymes 19
sterilization of 72
Intestine/liver transplant 105, 125, 126
animal experiments 106
basic considerations 106
clinical experience 107
comparison with isolated small bowel 108, 127
GVHD in 94
historical cases 107
postoperative 108
Intra-cytoplasmic brush-border enzymes 33
Intravenous fluids
following resection 3
Irradiation
enteropathy following 91
pretreatment with 38, 90, 124, 128
preventing GVHD 79
Isolated small bowel transplant 121–5
comparison with intestinal/liver transplant 108, 127
historical cases 112

Jejunal resection
with intact ileum and colon 5
Jejunum
absorption in 1
in celiac disease 59

D-Lactic acidosis 3
Liver
immunological protection from 107
role in intestinal grafting 101–11
tolerogenicity 106
with intestinal transplant
See Intestine/liver transplant
Lupus erythematosus 44
Lymphatic regeneration 24
Lymphocytes
B lymphocytes 31
in Peyer's patches 89
divisions of 44
in Peyer's patches 57
intraepithelial 57
NK lymphocytes 34
helper T lymphocytes 34, 51
radio-sensitive 91
rejection and 30

replacing graft cells 32
T lymphocytes 30, 34, 83
independent antigen 50
in GVHD 34, 38
mediated immunity 63
proliferation triggering 30
two-signal process 89
Lymphocytotoxic drug pretreatment 92
Lymphokines 30
damage by 133
release of 115, 116
signals 83
Lymphoma 129
Lysozyme in mucosal barrier 54

Macrophages
in lamina propria 33
in rejection 116
Major histocompatibility barriers 78
Major histocompatibility complex 88
antigen expression 90
incompatibility 89
Malnutrition 2
bacterial translocation and 63
Maltase
detection of 33
Maltose absorption 14, 15
in rejection 14, 15
in transplant 23
6-Mercapturine 122
Mesenteric lymphadenectomy 38, 93
Mesenteric plexus
regulating motility 25
Mesenteric thrombosis 126
Mesenteric vein in drainage 105
Methotrexate 92
Methylprednisolone 92, 123
Microchimerism 106
Mixed leukocyte reaction 88
Monoclonal antibodies
potency of 95
immunosuppression by 112
pretreatment with 94, 95
use of 32, 35
Monocyte procoagulant activity 34
Motility
experimental assessment 25
in normal intestine 25
regulation by myenteric plexus 25
transplantation 26
Mucin 56
Mucosa
exposure of 53
Mucosal barrier 53–69
bacterial translocation and 60–3, 65–6
components of 54
endotoxin and 66
function of 53
gastric acidity and 55
immaturity of function 53
loss of function 72
mucus in 56, 65
neonatal 53, 55, 56, 61
peristalsis and 64, 65
permeability and 57–60
proteolysis in 55
role of peristalsis 55
in small bowel transplantation 63
sugars crossing 59
Mucosal biopsies 33
Mucosal destruction 31
Mucosal immunity 43–52
in normal small bowel 43
Mucosal pattern in rejection 113
Mucus
in mucosal barrier 56, 65
Multivisceral transplantation 107, 125

Necrotizing enterocolitis 53, 54
Neonate
immaturity of stomach 55
mucosal barrier in 53, 55, 56, 57
Nutrient absorption 2
Nutritional failure 3
Nutritional requirements
in home parenteral nutrition 6

OKT 3
treat rejection with 108, 124, 127
deplete donor graft lymphocytes with 125
Oral feeding
after resection 4
Orthotopic grafts 11, 12, 20
function after 15

Pancreatic allografts 95
Pancreatico-duodenal transplant 125
Pancreatic proteases 71
Parenteral nutrition 4
home 5, 6, 118
Passenger leukocyte theory 88
Pathology of transplantation 112
Peptic ulceration
resection causing 3
Peristalsis 25
hyperactive 26
mucosal barrier and 55, 64, 65
in rejection 34
Peyer's patches 57, 61, 78
antigen-presenting cells in 89
M cells in 44, 57
graft cells in 35
Ia positive lymphoid cells in 95
immunoblast migration from 32
lymphocytes in 43, 57
T lymphocytes in 116

Polypeptides in intestine 19
Popliteal lymph node assay 37
Portal circulation
  in intestinal grafting 101–11
Portal diversion
  liver abnormality 102
Portal vein
  antigen infusion in 102
Portal venous drainage 12, 25, 105, 128
Prednisolone 81
Preservation of graft 70–7, 128
  cold storage affecting 71
  effect on histology 113
  epithelial damage from 74
  future prospects 133
  histological assessment 73–4
  ischaemia and 70
  pancreatic proteases and 71
  reperfusion injury 71, 75
  solutions 71, 72–3, 75
Pretreatment 78–9, 128
  antilymphocyte serum in 79, 81, 93, 124
  clinical considerations 96
  cyclosporin in 93, 94, 96
  disadvantages of radiation 91
  donor modification 89
  FK 506 93, 96
  immunotoxin perfusion 94
  irradiation 90, 91, 124, 128
  lymphocytoxic drugs 92
  mesenteric lymphadenectomy 93
  monoclonal antibodies 94, 95
  passenger leukocyte theory 88
  ultraviolet radiation 92
Procoagulant factor 129
Prostaglandin E_1 127, 134
Protein-losing enteropathy 114
Protein metabolism in intestine 19
Proteolysis in mucosal barrier 55

RS-61443 88
Radiation enteropathy 91
Raffinose in preservation 73
Rapamycin 88
  effect on graft survival 84
  treatment of recipients 83
Rat models 10, 18
  advantages of 11
  bacterial translocation in 66
  donor and graft irradiation 90
  intestine/liver transplant 106
  pretreatment in 93
  rejection in 31
Rejection 30–42, 127, 128, 129
  acute 31, 113
  in animal species 31
  biopsy in 114, 116, 129
  chronic 116
  clinical signs 113
  contact between graft and host antigens 30
  diagnosis of 32, 33, 112, 113–14
  early 115
  effect of immunosuppression on 32
  equilibrium with GVHD 34, 39
  experimental models 12, 13, 14
  histology of 114
  host sensitization in 30
  immunohistochemistry 114
  influence of venous drainage on 12
  in intestine/liver transplant 108
  maltose absorption and 15
  mucosal pattern in 113
  peristalsis in 34
  signs and symptoms 14
  timing of 115
  villus sloughing in 31, 32
Renal stones after resection 3

Saliva in mucosal barrier 54
Selective gut decontamination 63
Sepsis 129
  complicating home parenteral nutrition 6
Septic shock 113
Short bowel syndrome 15, 127
Skin changes in GVHD 34
Small bowel syndrome 1, 61, 124
Small bowel transplant *See under Intestinal transplant*
Sodium absorption in graft 21
Somatostatin analogue 5
Splanchic venous diversion 102
Spleen weight in GVHD 37
Steatorrhoea 2
Sugars
  crossing mucosal barrier 59

Thiry-Vella loop 9, 10, 21, 26
Tissue matching 134
Total parenteral nutrition 61
Translocation of bacteria
  See Bacterial translocation
Transplantation
  effect on physiology 18
  function of 12
  See also under Intestine etc
Trauma
  sepsis and 60
Triglycerides
  malabsorption of 4
Trinitrophenol-lipopolysaccharide 50
Tumour necrosis factor 116

Ultra-violet radiation
  in pretreatment 92
University of Wisconsin solution 72, 75, 113, 127, 128, 133
Urea synthesis in liver 102

Vascular reconstruction 128
Vasoactive intestinal polypeptide 70
Venous access in home parenteral nutrition 5
Venous drainage
  effect on rejection 12
  importance of 25
Venous outflow 101, 109
  from transplant 10
Villikinin 25
Villus
  motility 25
  oedema 114
  preservation damaging 74
  sloughing of tips 31, 32
  shortening in GVHD 34
Vitamin B
  absorption of 2, 4, 129
Vomiting in rejection 116

Water absorption
  in transplant 22
  in graft 21, 22
  through intestine 19

Xanthine oxidase reaction 58, 61, 71